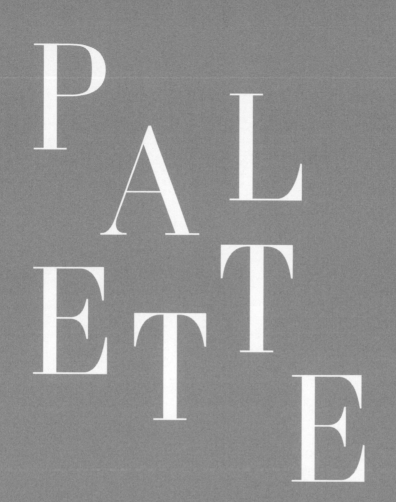

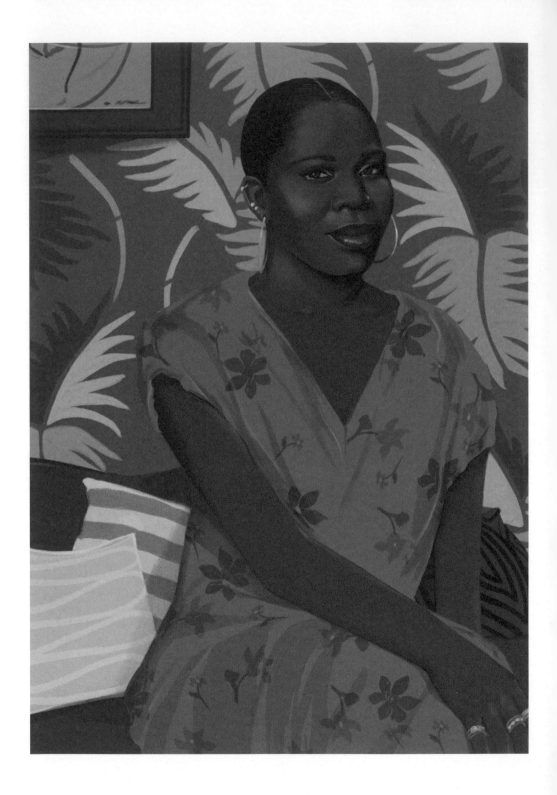

FUNMI FETTO is Executive Editor and Beauty
Director at *Glamour*, a columnist for the *Observer*
newspaper and a former beauty editor at British *Vogue*
where she also wrote a beauty column aimed at women
of colour. In her 20 years' experience as a fashion and
beauty journalist, she has also written and worked for
numerous publications including *The Sunday Times*,
Harper's Bazaar, *Guardian*, *Elle*, *Marie Claire* and
Tatler. Funmi Fetto also consults for and has worked
with a wide variety of global beauty brands and has
spoken on numerous panels covering topics relating to
beauty, identity, race and journalism.

The BEAUTY BIBLE
for WOMEN
of COLOUR

PALETTE

FUNMI FETTO

Illustrations by SPIROS HALARIS

CORONET

First published in Great Britain in 2019 by Coronet
An Imprint of Hodder & Stoughton
An Hachette UK company

1

Copyright © Funmi Fetto 2019

The right of Funmi Fetto to be identified as the Author of the Work has been asserted by her
in accordance with the Copyright, Designs and Patents Act 1988.

All illustrations by Spiros Halaris © Hodder & Stoughton, 2019
www.spiroshalaris.com

Design and art direction by Alice Laurent
www.aka-alice.co.uk

A CIP catalogue record for this title is available from the British Library

Hardback ISBN 978 1 529 33043 4
eBook ISBN 978 1 529 33047 2

Typeset in OL America The Beautiful by Dennis Ortiz-Lopez and Miller Text by Matthew Carter,
from Carter & Cone.

Printed and bound in Italy by Lego SpA

Hodder & Stoughton policy is to use papers that are natural, renewable and recyclable products
and made from wood grown in sustainable forests. The logging and manufacturing processes are
expected to conform to the environmental regulations of the country of origin.

Hodder & Stoughton Ltd
Carmelite House
50 Victoria Embankment
London EC4Y 0DZ

www.hodder.co.uk

To every woman of colour. This is for us.

In February 2017, to coincide with Black History Month in the United States, CNN launched a project inspired by W.E.B. Du Bois's *The Souls of Black Folk*, a literary classic about race and ethnicity in North America. In this book, Du Bois talks about the first time he realised that his skin colour made him different. CNN chronicled several high-profile people of colour revealing their own personal 'moment'. It was called 'The First Time I Realised I Was Black', and it was something I had never thought about. As I mulled over how I would respond, I had a realisation that it came back to beauty.

I was born in London; however, when I was five years old, we moved to Lagos, Nigeria. Here, the concept of 'Being Black' was irrelevant. We were Nigerians, we were Africans, and we were too preoccupied with class to fit in a conversation about what it meant to be black. I came back to London when I was ten. That first day back at school, I knew I was different. I had a short Afro, and I remember overhearing a comment about me looking like Kunta Kinte, the character in Alex Haley's novel *Roots* who was captured from his African village and sold into slavery. During swimming class, there was another comment that my 'rubber lips' should keep me afloat.

These remarks made me realise I was different, but they didn't make me think about being black. As I hit adolescence, I began to get interested in beauty. I would, surreptitiously, take one of my mother's lipsticks and swipe it across my lips as I walked to school, hoping to come across as worldly and sophisticated. One day, I went into a local chemist with some Caucasian friends to check out the beauty offering. While my friends giggled excitedly about their finds, everything I tried either left an ashy finish or didn't show up on my skin because the pigments were not strong enough. Still I persevered, desperate to be part of the collective. I tried on the darkest foundation; a shade called Biscuit. To hide my embarrassment, I laughed off the fact that I looked as if I had smeared chalk on my skin.

But, of course, at that moment, everything changed. Suddenly colour mattered, in more ways than one. This is when I first realised I was 'black'. It was as if I had turned up at an exclusive private party, to which I was not invited. I felt irrelevant, excluded and ashamed. I was not valuable enough to be part of the beauty conversation.

That experience was a few decades ago but, inconceivably, even with the world's best beauty products at my disposal, I continue to relive that Biscuit moment. For years, the beauty industry peddled the 'Black Doesn't Sell' myth. I attend hair launches, where the products are all about getting swishy 'French-girl hair'. 'Global' skincare launches, where the 'extensive product testing' has only been conducted on white women. Launches where a make-up artist is giving everyone a makeover but doesn't have your shade. Events where raising your hand to question the inclusivity of the products on show is met with an exasperated eye roll by other members of the media. And then there are the 'nude' lipstick launches, where the range would struggle to suit anyone darker than the colour of, yes, a biscuit.

As a beauty journalist who is sent products every month, I can test things and find out what will work for my skin and hair. But what about all the other women of colour out there? For years, strangers, colleagues, friends, family – in the street, at dinner parties, via social media – have been asking me for advice. 'What's the best foundation for oily skin?', 'What works well on hyperpigmentation?', 'Does that new brand everyone is raving about on Instagram work on us?', 'What do you think about coconut oil for natural hair?', 'Do I need retinol?'

Women of colour want to be able to walk into any mainstream store selling beauty products and buy haircare, skincare and cosmetics without a second thought. As an industry, we are moving in the right direction, but there is still a lot of work to be done. This is what inspired me to write *Palette*.

For every woman of colour on the hunt for beauty products that speak to her, this book is for you. It is also a rallying cry for all beauty brands to recognise the necessity, importance and value of engaging with a diverse range of skin tones and hair textures. Let's banish the Biscuit experience for good.

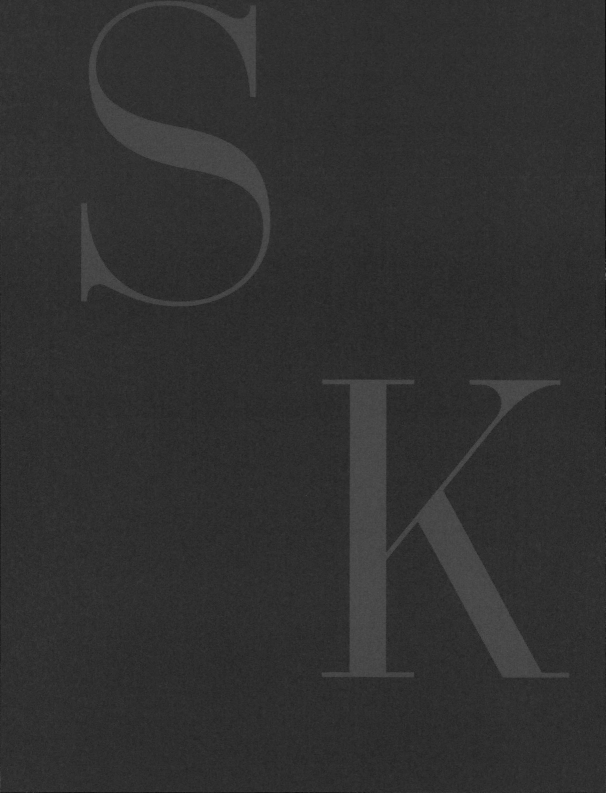

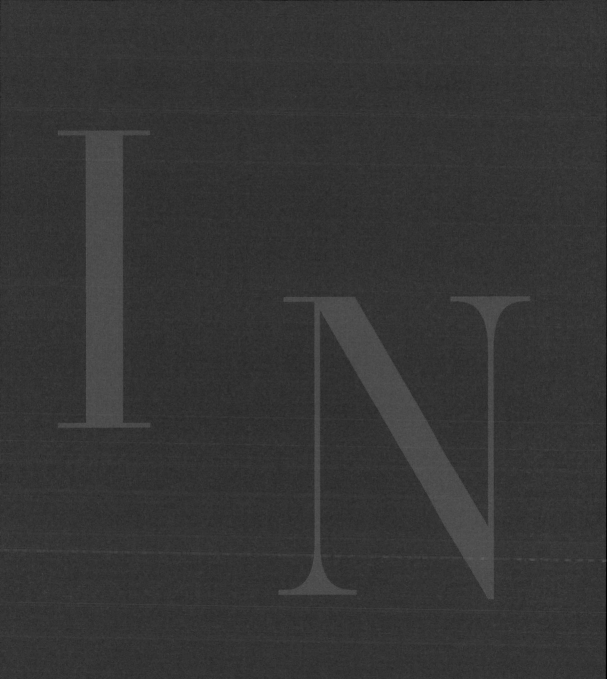

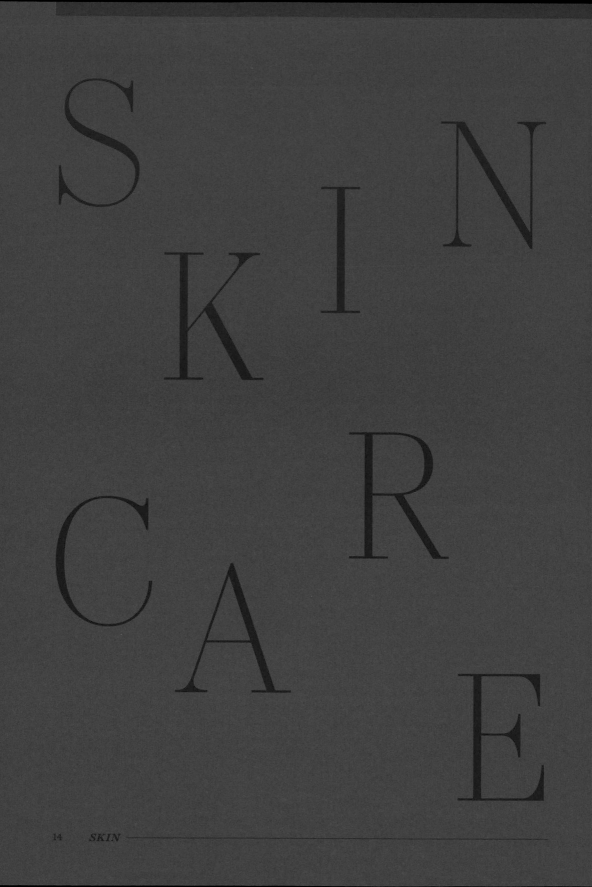

SKIN CARE

A h, the irony. Here I am writing about skincare, and my skin is the worst it has been in a while. But please don't let that put you off. Here's the thing, unless you have perfect genes, chances are that you will, at some point, face some challenges to your skin because, you know what? Life happens. Life for me, at the moment, means being a self-appointed guinea pig. I am trying and retrying new products and old favourites for the sake of this book, and this can play havoc with your skin. Think of me as the martyr who has been to Calvary and back for the sake of everyone's skin salvation. (The lesson here? All the products in this book are great; just don't use them all at once.)

As someone who suffered from terrible skin for many years – breakouts, acne, pigmentation, uneven texture, you name it – it is a blessing to have a job where I can access the knowledge I need to get my skin to a place where I am happy to go out without make-up. (And I mean properly out – not just out as in 'putting the bins out'). Why wouldn't I want to share that with you? I've said, and I will keep saying, in the hope that brands will listen, that there are products out there that work for us, but if we are not represented or included in the marketing then how are we supposed to know?

While reading this book, please bear the following in mind:

When choosing a product, ask yourself this: would you invest in the same outfit for a funeral, for the beach, for raving at Afropunk and for a traditional wedding? No, you wouldn't. The point? Context is key. You cannot expect a single product to work for every eventuality.

I remember meeting a woman of colour (a facialist) with skin so marble smooth you could roll puff pastry on it. She admitted that she never used any of the products she was about to use on me (which naturally filled me with great confidence); all she ever used was Vaseline. Now, if I slathered my face in Vaseline, my skin would give birth to aliens. Not every product works for everyone. You have to find what's right for you.

There are, however, three things that I believe every woman of colour should have in her skincare repertoire. First, a liquid exfoliator: this will give your skin LIFE. Second, vitamin C in some form, or another kind of brightener. Please understand that I am not talking about bleaching here, I'm talking about something to tackle those pesky dark spots and keep pigmentation at bay. And then, finally, sunscreen. Without sunscreen, all your hard work will go to the dogs.

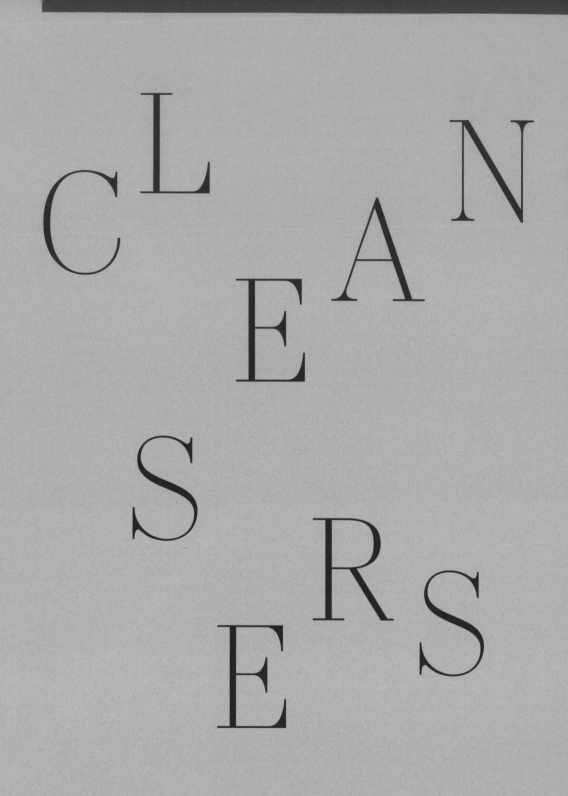

CLEANSERS

THINGS TO NOTE...

Cleansers can no longer expect a round of applause just because they clean. That's the bare minimum, so put them through their paces and expect more from yours. Your texture of choice is down to personal preference, but if you have blemished, oily skin, and choose a rich balm that promises to hydrate dry skin, it won't do a thing for you. Identify what your skin needs and choose your product accordingly.

NIOD
Sanskrit Saponins

Is it a bird? Is it a plane? Is it a ...? Exactly. My first thought when I came across Sanskrit Saponins was 'what on earth is this?' Trying to unravel the nature of a product with only a double-Dutch press release and some Google search results that would send even the most learned specialist spiralling into a state of panic, always feels like a little too much work. Especially when you are on deadline. But then two things happened. First, I noticed an influx of this type of 'intellectual skincare', a burgeoning movement of product ranges that most people would need a medical degree to decipher. And second, my face wash ran out. Why not try the crazy-sounding cleanser? I was blown away. The brand blurb is that it helps to remove dead skin cells and reduces the look of pores while also combating blemishes and congestion. Quite a tall order, but SS does everything it says on the tin and more – you notice a difference on first use. It gets rid of deep-rooted gunk, so you end up with incredibly clean skin and a beautifully smooth texture. Unlike most deep cleans, it does not mess up the pH balance of your skin, so you don't have that 'if I smile my face will crack' feeling. It is utterly brilliant. You're advised to use SS every other day. I personally think that depends on two things: your skin type (sensitive and dry skins may need to go easy) and your skin's reaction. I have oily skin so used it every day and the only reaction I had was better skin. The texture is quite strange – creamy, milky, ever so slightly foamy, all at the same time. And the smell is also slightly odd – a little bit like yeast mixed with fertiliser. Not disgusting, but it's there. Still, considering the results, it's a small price to pay.

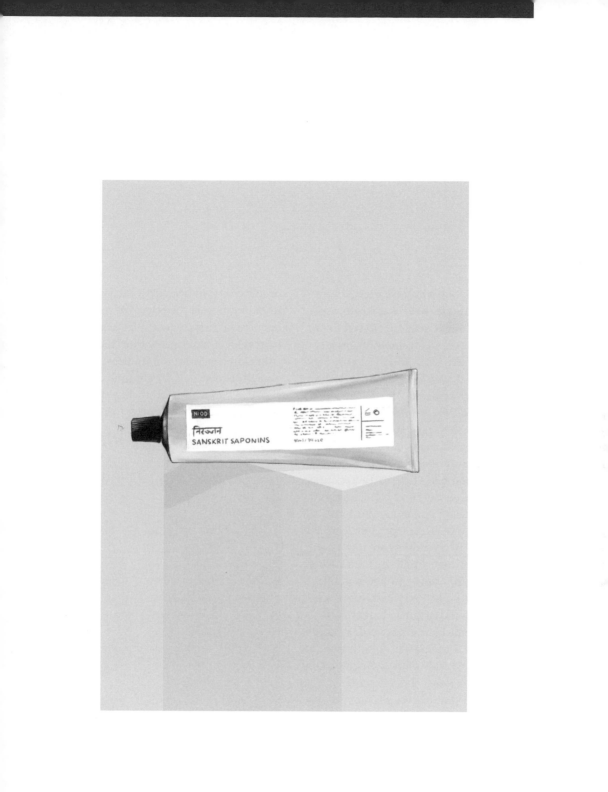

SUNDAY RILEY
Ceramic Slip

Nearly everyone who gave me a 5-star review of this cleanser was white, and for a long time, it never occurred to me to try it. Also, if I hear something is a 'gentle' cleanser, what I really hear is 'Hey guys, I don't do very much'. But curiosity got the better of me, so I tried a recently reformulated Ceramic Slip. I never used the old formula (there is a raging argument in the beauty world as to which is best), but I can tell you, this product is phenomenal. As someone who has long battled oiliness, blemishes, breakouts and pigmentation issues (as a teen I remember thinking, 'Life, you have FAILED me') I have to force myself to try products that are not just about dealing with those issues. There are always other things to consider, like hydration or protecting the skin barrier, and these, in the end, help to rectify the other problems like oiliness and breakouts. That is what Ceramic Slip does. It is a silky gel formulated with a blend of plant-based soaps, French green clay, bentonite and white kaolin clay. It gives you a really deep clean but it does so without drying the skin. Antioxidant-rich and skin-balancing ingredients such as olive oil and rice esters have been incorporated into the formula to protect the skin from dehydration. But more than that, it gets the grime off your skin and out of your pores – gently. It doesn't take long at all before you see that the texture of your skin has improved immeasurably and everything feels more balanced. A lesson in how to cleanse your face brilliantly without beating it into submission.

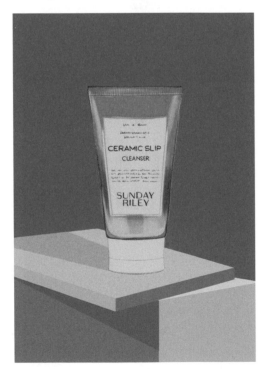

PETER THOMAS ROTH
Anti-Aging Cleansing Gel

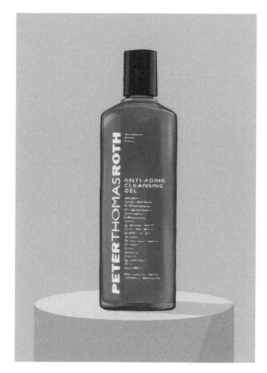

In many 'safe space' beauty confessional moments, women sheepishly admit to me that they have, on more than the odd occasion, gone to bed with a full face of make-up still on. It takes the love of God for me not to shudder and recoil in judgement. I don't go to bed with my make-up on – the idea that the day's debris would be left to fester and have a rave in my pores fills me with terror – but I have, of course, been tempted. For the most part, the temptation comes when I am utterly exhausted. At moments like this, if I could employ someone to wash my face, I most definitely would. The more reasonable alternative to this is Peter Thomas Roth Anti-Aging Cleansing Gel. In some ways you could say it is the J-Lo of cleansers – it excels in a bit of everything and gives good glow. As a deep cleanser, it makes a difference that is akin to a facial and the longer you use it, the more you'll notice the benefits. The texture is a light gel that on contact with water produces suds (more 'light, creamy shaving foam' than 'bubble bath', and you won't go blind if they get in your eyes); that clear out any build-up in your pores, lift your make-up straight off and treat breakouts, while simultaneously staving them off (that's the salicylic acid in the formulation). The citrus fruits and white-oak-bark extracts brighten the skin, and the glycolic acid refines the texture. This makes it perfect for those with pigmentation and breakout issues, though not appropriate for sensitive-skin types (try their **Water Drench® Cloud Cream Cleanser** instead). For everyone else, I would suggest starting off by alternating this with something more hydrating and see how your face fares with the acids. Now, will you please stop going to bed with your make-up on?

BIOLOGIQUE RECHERCHE
Lait VIP O$_2$

My introduction to Biologique Recherche, an exclusive, bespoke French skincare range did not bode well. This brand has had cult status for many years and industry insiders swear by it. I was intrigued and wanted to know more, but soon discovered that the website had no prices and didn't allow you to purchase the products. That irritated me. I asked the press office for products to try so I could write about them. I was told I would need to come in for an initial bespoke skin analysis (which you can now do online) before I could get hold of anything. Admittedly, the product labels were in French and had a bewildering numbering system – P50, P400, MC110 – which may as well have been tax codes. I was time and patience poor, and the thought of traipsing to a clinic on the other side of London was exasperating. And so, irritated at what I deemed an unnecessary preciousness, I dismissed BR, consoling myself that since all those rhapsodising about its greatness were Caucasian, it probably wasn't for me anyway.

Years later, I was invited to have a Biologique Recherche facial at Liberty. Just 60 minutes later, every adjective I could use to describe my face ended in 'er': better, cleaner, clearer, plumper, brighter, glowier ... you get the gist. Unsurprisingly, I did a shameless U-turn and set about using the BR skincare line. On opening the bag of samples I was sent home with, the waft that hit me was clinical and nauseating. At best it reminded me of the sick bay at school; at worst, of a time I spent in hospital in Lagos recovering from malaria. Still I persevered and discovered this milky cleanser to be a triumph. Oh, the fabulous texture! It is the cleanser version of a dulcet tone: super silky, creamy, and so smooth. It feels heavenly to use, like cleansing with a thick, rich night cream that leaves the skin hydrated and balanced without any stickiness. It contains an impressive oxygenating complex that enhances oxygen delivery, and the more oxygen your skin has, the better your skincare products will work. It also filters out pollution, so is particularly good for urbanites, and removes make-up without traumatising your skin. Would I make a beeline for this if I wanted something specifically for pigmentation and/or acne-prone skin? No. It makes sense to choose your cleanser according to your pressing needs – I wouldn't go into a taxidermist looking for a vegan dessert. Ultimately, what Lait VIP O_2 does is give you a better version of the skin you have. But you still can't just walk into a shop and buy it. An irritation I just have to live with.

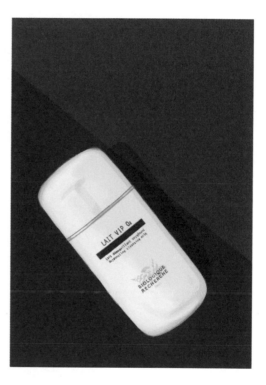

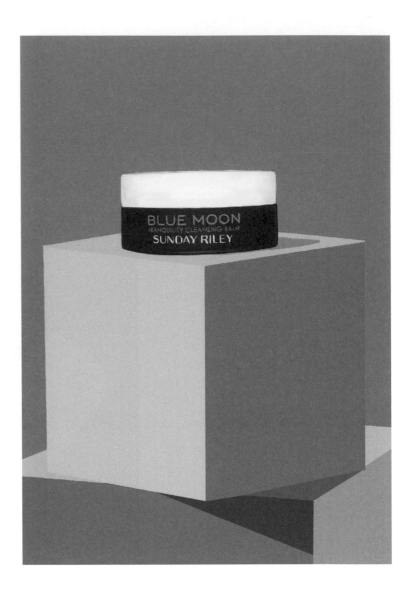

SUNDAY RILEY
Blue Moon Tranquility Cleansing Balm

The week I tried this – an unctuous cornflower-blue balm filled with very fine, barely there sugar grains – was also the week I had given up sugar (I find not eating sugar gets rid of and prevents me from getting breakouts). It was also the week I was dreaming of owning the opening look from a recent Valentino catwalk show – an incredible pleated dress the same shade as this cleanser but at a price point that would give my bank balance an allergic reaction. I suppose you could say that this cleanser was a roundabout way of satisfying my cravings. The light scent (cocoa butter, tangerine and sweet-orange essential oils) was a lovely, surprising opener. In a time when everyone is preaching the benefits of fragrance free, this mindset may seem slightly out of touch, but let's not deny the importance of the sensorial aspect of skincare. The balm turns to a gorgeous milky texture that leaves skin hydrated and soothed. You need only a tiny amount, but you will also need to double cleanse in order to remove really heavy make-up. And even then, it leaves a little something on your skin. Not make-up or dirt residue, more of a 'Oooh, great, I don't need anything else' type residue. This is wonderful if you see the Korean beauty 10-step skincare routine as masochistic but not if you relish a multistep regime. For oilier skin types, though, this is potentially too rich. It works much more effectively on sensitive, drier, more mature skins and if you like multi-tasking products, this is a no-brainer. Yes, there are now numerous products that promise to clean, exfoliate and moisturise. Most are a disaster. This one doesn't actually sell itself as a polymath as such, but it does deliver. Not quite the sugar fix or the Valentino dress I'd really like, but, for now, I'll live vicariously through it.

MURAD
Environmental Shield
Essential-C Cleanser

The nature of my job is such that I am constantly rotating my products and treatments. There is an upside to this: I get to discover and explore a deluge of products I never would have come across or even considered using. This hopefully makes me better at my job. The downside, however, is that there are times I am so keen on discovering the new that I forget the old. I flirt with and fall for inappropriate suitors, but then run back to my ex when things go horribly wrong, crying 'Why did I ever leave you?' This sums up my relationship with Murad's Environmental Shield Essential-C Cleanser. Unlike many beauty products, whose formulations are constantly being altered (mostly at their peril), this cleanser, a citrusy antioxidant gel, has stayed consistent in its brilliance. The 'C' in the title is vitamin C, which is incredibly brightening and targets uneven skin tones. It is also anti-pollution, meaning it combats the effects of environmental aggressors (smoke, air conditioning, general pollution), and it cleans deeply but gently. I love that it is austerity conscious so you get a lot for your buck. For the plethora of women dealing with issues such as hyperpigmentation and overproduction of sebum, I would go as far as to say that it will transform your skin – it did mine – particularly when used in conjunction with **Murad Environmental Shield Essential-C Toner** (I don't generally like toners but, goodness, that product is next level magic). So now when anyone, exhausted from navigating the overwhelming complexities of beauty products, asks me to recommend a straightforward, good-value uncomplicated cleanser, this is the one I automatically endorse. And, before you ask, no, I don't have shares in it. But I probably should.

EVE LOM
Cleanser

Many moons ago I was interning at a fashion magazine but had applied for a proper assistant job at another publication. It was a bona-fide job that paid real-life money, still shockingly low but unlike the non-existent intern salary, afforded me the luxury of eating and not being evicted. I was down to the last two candidates, then got the call: I was not the chosen one. That same day I also had an appointment to review an Eve Lom facial. I was deflated by the rejection and had completely lost interest in going, but I'd given my word, and so off I went, head slumped, fighting the urge to scream, 'Why not me?!!!' What took place in the next two hours not only changed my mood, but totally changed my skin too. All Eve Lom used was this thick, balmy cleanser, which she massaged vigorously all over my face. By the time I left, I was totally indifferent to my earlier rejection and despite not having a scrap of make-up on, brimming with new-found confidence. To put this in context, I had long struggled with acne-prone, hyperpigmented skin, and the idea of not hiding my face and skin under a huge weave or thick foundation was alien to me. After consistently using this cleanser at home (with the accompanying exfoliating muslin cloths), my skin was clearer (the balm draws out the toxins) and more balanced (my greasy T-zone calmed right down), my face less puffy (the massaging – SO key – it helps with lymphatic drainage), and blackheads that had been hovering under my skin for years finally made an exit. This is how my love affair with Eve Lom's cleanser began. Unsurprisingly, it is one of those beauty products that has cult-classic status. It really does improve the quality of all skin texture. Despite this, I know SO many people who hate it. A handful of friends complain about the balmy texture. Many take offence at the smell, because key ingredients include hops (the yeasty stuff with which you flavour beer), eucalyptus and clove oils. If you think those scents are likely to make you heave, I still urge you to give it a try. It might be worth it for the sake of decent skin. Personally, I have no issue with the smell. It might be that my olfactory organs were indoctrinated by that first remarkable encounter. And the fact that, a few months later, I was offered a full-time fashion-assistant role at *Harper's Bazaar*. Result, on every level.

DR BARBARA STURM
Darker Skin Tones
Enzyme Cleanser

Years ago, when I was invited for a one to one meeting with Dr Barbara Sturm I jumped at the chance for a three reasons. First, she's the German cosmetics doctor loved by Hollywood and famed for the Vampire Facial – it involves extracting a patient's blood, separating the plasma, rich in growth factors, and then injecting it back into the face. Her clientele think this is totally normal. Second, she was launching a new skincare line aimed at darker skin tones and the packaging wasn't all garish colours with a picture of an overly airbrushed woman wearing a bottomless weave and a ludicrous facial expression. Third, she had developed the line with the actress Angela Bassett, and Angela Bassett was going to be joining us. IN. THE. FLESH. How could I resist? I met Dr Barbara and found her to be an exceptionally brilliant, forward-thinking scientist worth her salt. And then Angela – elegant, kind, charming and just divine. But more than that, her skin was flawless. This she attributed to Dr Barbara Sturm, so I didn't need much more convincing.

For me everything starts with a great cleanser, but when I eagerly opened the box, I did wonder whether I had mistakenly been given an empty sample – the bottle was feather light. I quickly realized that it contained a powder made up of vitamin C and enzymes, and that these granules work to loosen the glue that holds dead skin cells together. It reminds me a little of the old-school Japanese washing grains I used to buy years ago – I was a sucker for anything that promised to give me decent skin – except this actually works. You pour a little of the powder into your palm, mix with warm water and make a paste. You massage the thin creamy paste into your face and rinse it off. Straight away your skin looks cleaner (I say that because there are cleansers that are rubbish at cleaning), smoother (this is perfect for reducing sebum production and oiliness, without stripping) and brighter (that's the vitamin C at work). The paste-making situation sounds like a faff, but it isn't. It also works as a peel, but unlike other peels, there's no tingling (I can hear the reverberating echoes of AMEN from all those with an aversion to discomfort). It has no scent or hue to speak of; the packaging is not terribly exciting. There's no singing, no dancing, no nothing. But as a cleanser – and, ultimately, this is what counts – it is genius: superb in its functionality and excellent value for money.

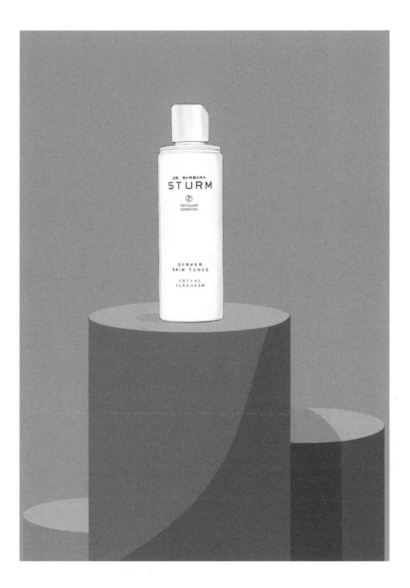

Good ski
like love,
have to h
can tingle
burns, it's

care,
oesn't
rt. It
but if it
no good.

KIEHL'S
Midnight Recovery
Botanical Cleansing Oil

I love how this smells. I have bemoaned the fact that the obsession with fragrance free is killing one of the primary pleasures of skincare. Of course, if anything smells artificial, overpowering or remotely gourmand (ugh, please don't get me started), I run a mile. But this cult favourite is a fine balance, and incidentally that's what the product does – it balances out the skin and helps it retain its natural moisture levels. It is non-comedogenic (so won't clog your pores), sulphate free and mineral-oil free. One oil it does include is squalane, an old-school ingredient that has recently become fashionable again because it helps to prevent loss of hydration and increases skin suppleness. Brilliant for all skin types, but especially appealing to more mature skin. The brand pitches this as a product best used at night. Mostly I dismiss this type of instruction as marketing blurb, but, in this scenario, it is worth paying attention to.

Sure, the world won't come to an end if you use it in the morning, but I have found it to be more effective at bedtime as it gives you the added hydration and moisture needed at night – particularly during winter. It also has calming aromatherapy properties (evening primrose and lavender essential oils) perfect for aiding sleep, a little unhelpful on Monday mornings. For me, however, the best thing about this product is that it meets a fundamental need. It takes off your make-up – quickly: yes, even cloggy mascara. Anything that means I don't wake up with panda eyes and unyielding black stains on my pillow gets my vote every time.

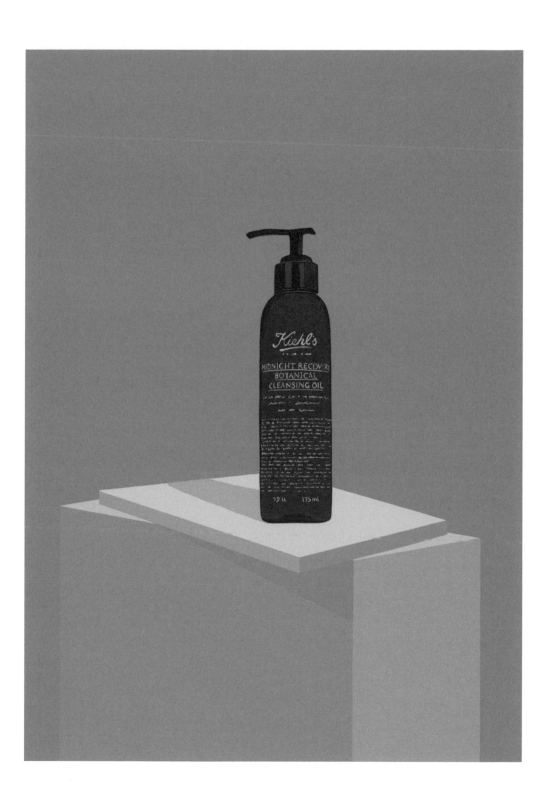

THE INKEY LIST™
Salicylic Acid Cleanser

You see that bonkers list of ingredients on the back of your beauty product? That is known as the International Nomenclature of Cosmetic Ingredients (INCI) list, and on some products, it can induce a migraine if you try to understand it. Colette Newberry and Mark Curry decided to launch a single-ingredient brand that anyone could understand without being a chemistry boffin. It's called The Inkey List (get it?), and it is the epitome of hi–lo beauty; that is, high quality, low price. Admittedly, the packaging doesn't float my boat, but it's priced reasonably and does a pretty awesome job. I can always happily kick my design snobbery to the curb for the sake of an efficacious product. I am pretty diligent with my skincare regime – yes, it's a regime; what, you think I do the 10-step routine because I love it? – however, there was a point where, regardless of what I put on my skin, breakouts refused to leave. This cleanser, a combination of salicylic acid (an exfoliator that removes debris from the skin and pores), zinc (great for controlling sebum production) and allantoin (an anti-irritant) changed my skin almost overnight. It also costs less than my weekly coffee splurge, which was probably what caused me to break out in the first place. But we can just ignore that bit.

DRUNK ELEPHANT™
Pekee Bar™

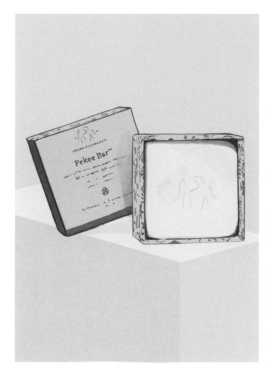

I am inexplicably obsessed with luxe bar soaps, but somewhat ridiculously, I rarely use them. Instead, I treat soaps as you would collectables; stare at them, infatuated fangirl style, displayed and untouched like museum pieces. This adoration does not extend to bars of soap pitched for the face. I mean, as far as I'm concerned, you may as well wash your face with toilet cleaner. Or so I thought, until Drunk Elephant's Pekee Bar landed on my desk. For those who haven't heard of it, Drunk Elephant is the US-born clean-conscious, toxin-free brand we beauty editors have been obsessed with for years. Up until recently, however, it was only available in the States, and so every trip across the Atlantic would involve a requisite trip to Sephora for a haul. It is hyped up, Insta adored, beloved by beauty aficionados and has a very strong cult following. When it finally arrived in the UK, the industry went into a frenzy. The stars of this brand are some of the serums (**T.L.C. Framboos™ Glycolic Night Serum, C-Firma™ Day Serum**) and oils (**Virgin Marula Luxury Facial Oil**), but I think Pekee is the hidden gem (and, to boot, it is nowhere near as eye-wateringly expensive as the rest of the brand). It looks like a soap, it's shaped like a soap, and it smells like a soap but, technically, it is not a soap. Its PH level is a beautifully skin-balancing 6.51 (soap, on the other hand, is upwards of 9 – aka a skin-destroying beast). Expect Pekee's creamy lather to gift you with skin that is brighter, super hydrated and pore-degunking-ly clean. My only criticism is that it goes down quickly, which then makes it too thin to use effectively. Still, the fact that it doesn't leave your face tighter than Scrooge is good enough.

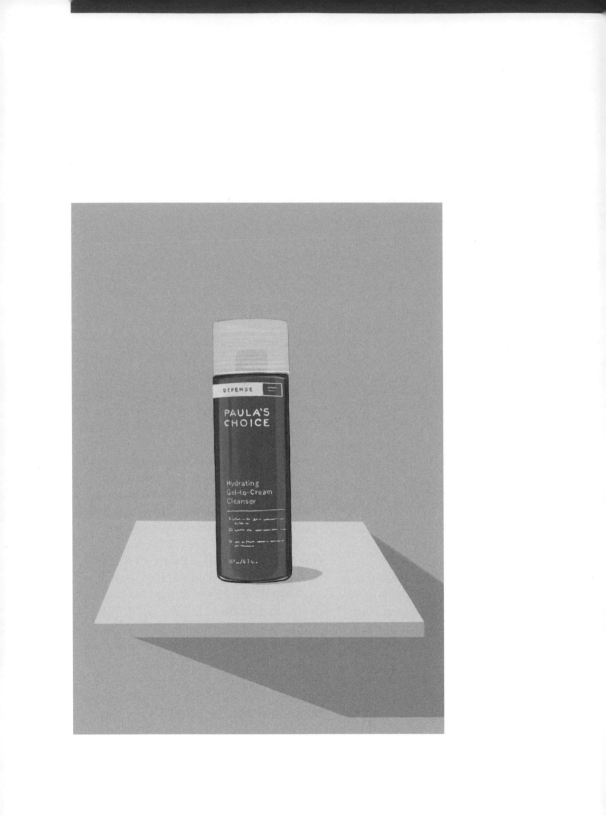

PAULA'S CHOICE
Hydrating Gel-to-Cream Cleanser

Years ago, I heard a high-profile dermatologist tut disapprovingly about how we – yes, all of us – are just not taking the time to wash our faces properly. (My immediate thought being, Oh, that's surprising. I mean, who revels in such a pedestrian act? Perhaps more people would spend extra time washing their faces if the ritual weren't so boring.) He went on to explain that the correct way to wash our faces is to leave the cleanser on for a little while, like you would a mask, and massage it in for a while longer to get the best results. And, of course, he's right. That little tweak in your routine is the one that will give you the best possible skin. But when you've had a long day, have an early start the next morning and live a high-pressured life, you are so close to the edge that all you want is something that washes your face in five minutes flat. Well, drum roll, here it is. I love Paula's

Choice as a brand. I find the formulations trustworthy, smart and grounded in science, and this new addition to the range does not disappoint. This is one of a new breed of 'easy' cleansers on the market, specifically developed to combat skin-damaging pollutants that prematurely age skin. The texture is a light, clear gel that turns creamy and lathers beautifully when watered. It very quickly but gently dissolves make-up, hydrates dry complexions, balances oily ones and cleans and softens skin in a way that is really quite phenomenal. You'll find your serums penetrate much better and your skin now looks so glowy that light bounces off it. I love the fact that it is so easy to use and delivers results quickly. It makes washing your face much less of a chore: a lazy girl's dream.

iS CLINICAL®
Cleansing Complex

This has been described as 'the ultimate cleansing formula'. High praise, indeed. Is it justified? Well, actually, it kind of is. There are a slew of cosmeceuticals (skincare brands with 'medical' benefits) on the market, many of which are quite hardcore. In my opinion, the 'no pain no gain' mantra is archaic. I don't believe your skin has to shed like a German Shepherd for it to look better. But iS Clinical is a different kind of skincare brand: gentle, but powerful – a bit like the Queen. This non-foaming gel combines antioxidants, salicylic and glycolic acids to address a number of skin issues. It gives your pores a deep clean (you can almost hear them breathing) and helps prevent breakouts, while also treating the blemishes that already exist. Your skin texture is resurfaced and looks more refined, vitamin C brightens and protects against free radicals, and the calming chamomile keeps irritation at bay. Now, let's be clear, this is maybe not a brand you would put on the Insta grid to celebrate its eye-candy worthiness. But what the packaging lacks in aesthetic appeal, it more than makes up for in its clever and efficacious approach to skincare. It is not a sexy brand; it is a brand that works.

RMK
Smooth Cleansing Oil

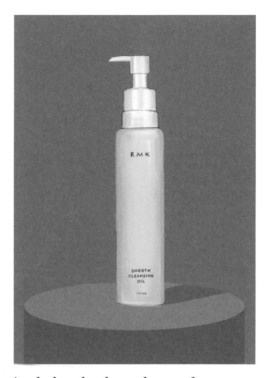

Pore clogger. Years ago, those were the words that came to mind when anyone suggested oil cleansers. And who could blame me? The term is such an oxymoron. The Japanese were way ahead of the game (they are responsible for bringing this cleansing formula to the West) and have long advocated oil cleansers as really gentle – but hugely effective – make-up removers, which are also stupendous at declogging and balancing the skin. And yet many I have tried are so basic in their formulation, I suspect they are no different from the vegetable oils I'd use to fry plantain. They leave a film on your skin and you wake up with breakouts. Needless to say, there are oil cleansers and then there are oil cleansers that work. RMK Smooth Cleansing Oil is the latter. I can't pinpoint when or even how I discovered this Japanese oil cleanser but once I did, I became obsessed. I would hunt it down – it was and still is not widely available – and I would bulk buy. Slightly scented – a pleasant citrusy mint – this superlight oil dissolves into a milky finish that exfoliates (with orange peel and carrot seed oils), removes surface and deep-rooted impurities and rinses off sans drama. The best thing about it is that skin feels really clean and balanced – not dry, not greasy, just hydrated and a good canvas for serums and moisturisers. Some people would encourage you to limit oils to the winter, but I find this is all down to your skin – I use it across the seasons and still get results. If you have an aversion to the smell of mint, you probably won't like this. If you prefer a thicker, heavier consistency (perhaps because you have more mature skin) then you won't like this. If you don't like oil cleansers, you won't like this. But if your priority is clean pores, hydrated and non-greasy skin, this will totally float your boat.

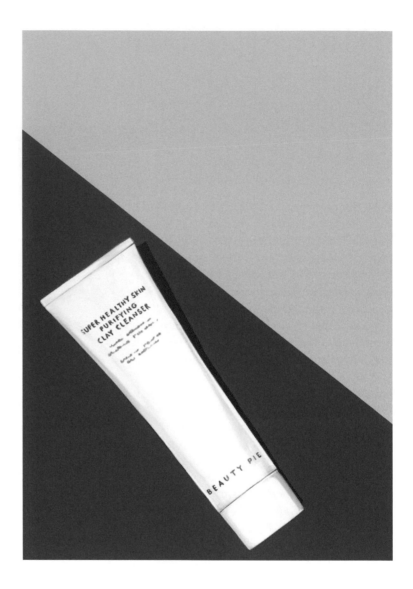

BEAUTY PIE™
Super Healthy Skin™
Deep Purifying Clay Cleanser

This paste – for that is what it is, a thick, velvety paste – has been described as 'a facial at your fingertips'. It doesn't behave in the way you expect a cleanser to. When it goes onto the skin, it is reminiscent of an old-school clay mask, without the inevitable drying and cracking. It is opaque in its whiteness and covers every crevice of your skin, leaving you resembling a ghoul. There's no tingling, no coolness, no heat, no tightness. Nothing. These days – particularly with product manufacturers yielding to our acid obsession – we are so accustomed to putting things on our faces that, rightly or wrongly, react on our skin in a certain way. That's our signal that something is happening. But with this you get a light-bulb moment only when you begin to wash it off. Your skin looks terrific afterwards. The formulation is understated but astute – the kaolin and montmorillonite (yes, it's a mouthful) clay detoxifies the pores and absorbs excess oil. There are acids (lactic, which exfoliates and smooths, lauric, which is a gentle cleanser), but you would only know this from the results. It is suitable for all, but particularly great for oilier skin types or those prone to breakouts. For even better results, use it with a cleansing brush – but nothing too harsh. Though I cannot imagine this cleanser antagonising skin, drier types may need to alternate with an equally gentle non-clay cleanser. While there are member and non-member prices for all the products (which are only available from their site), being a paid-up member of Beauty Pie makes decent financial sense as you will be able to purchase this for the price of a smoothie.

EXFOLIATORS

THINGS TO NOTE...

The liquid ones are a dream for your
face – they will make you look alive and
your skincare work harder than ever.
The ones containing those scratchy
particles are, generally, to be avoided.

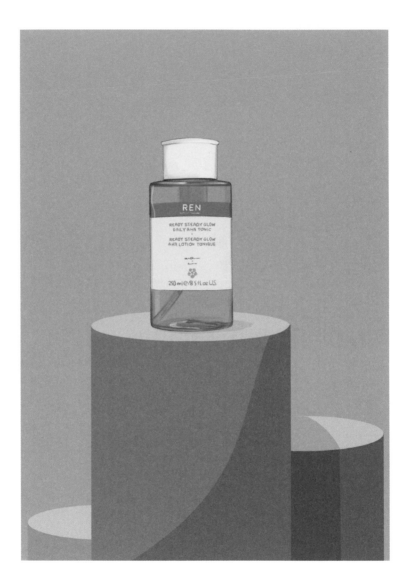

REN
Ready Steady Glow
Daily AHA Tonic

After so many years in this industry, one invariably develops what I see as a healthy dose of scepticism. I hold this mindset dear, otherwise I'd have been duped into thinking cellulite creams were worth the money, and Goop's Jade vaginal egg was a wonderful idea. This attitude, of course, has its downside; if you don't keep it in check, it can stop you from discovering something truly magnificent. Like this tonic right here. Prior to discovering this product, I had never used anything from REN. It is a brand well known for its clean, green and sustainable ethos. Perhaps it was the echo of voices in the beauty industry harping on about how wonderfully 'natural' it is that put me off. I had always associated those sorts of beauty products with a lack of grounding in science and an inability to deal with the issues that plague darker skin tones.

However, when this Glow Tonic came on the scene, I was (and still am) in full-on obsession mode with liquid exfoliators, and it smashed any preconceived ideas I had about the brand. This product,

a dead-skin-removing, brightening Alpha Hydroxy Acid (AHA) and Beta Hydroxy Acid (BHA) concoction, is incredible. It is where nature meets science to create something really brilliant – and at an affordable price point. The BHA is salicin, which exfoliates on a deeper level to detox your pores while preventing oiliness and breakouts, and the azelaic acid helps to even out the skin tone. The result is completely resurfaced, cleaner, brighter skin that glows. I would suggest starting by using it twice a week as it does tingle and takes some getting used to, particularly if you have sensitive skin. I use it daily, and I simply splash onto my face cologne style. You may get quicker results applying with a cotton pad, but if I'm too exhausted (aren't we all?) that just feels like an extra faff and, besides, this seems to work for me. To think I had almost written off REN. It's a lesson that reminded me of something I heard years ago: 'The most valuable thing to take with you when you go shopping is not your purse, it's an open mind.'

PAULA'S CHOICE
Skin Perfecting
2% BHA Liquid Exfoliant

The first time I met Paula Begoun, the walking beauty encyclopedia who founded the (since sold) Paula's Choice, I embarrassed myself. I became choked up as I told her how much this product had changed my skin and, therefore, my life. A force of nature – there isn't much about beauty, formulations and ingredients that this woman doesn't know – she also welled up in gratitude, which somewhat lessens the mortification I feel whenever I recall that moment.

This liquid exfoliator is possibly the product I have recommended the most to women everywhere. If there was ever an inkling that it might be discontinued, I would be thrown into chaos and take to the streets with a placard. It removes dead skin, gets rid of debris in the pores and refines my skin, making it smoother, more balanced and giving it a healthy glow. Thanks to the potency of the bacteria-busting salicylic acid, I am less likely to break out when using this. It also makes my make-up-free face look a million times better and acts as a great canvas under serums, sunscreen and make-up. I use it on my skin after my cleanser, splashing it on my face as if it is cologne, as opposed to using a cotton pad. Yes, I know a pad is more efficient, but I am convinced it sucks up more product than is absorbed into my skin, and encourages me to aggressively swipe across my face. That is totally unnecessary: this is a liquid exfoliator that doesn't need elbow grease to work. One thing to note – it comes in both a liquid and gel form, but I've found the liquid to be more effective, and best for oilier skins; the gel is best for drier skin types. The words 'game changer' are overused in the beauty industry, but, in this instance, they are fitting. This is the one beauty item I would insist on if I were banished to a desert island. Well, this and sunscreen – because nobody needs extra pigmentation problems.

DR DENNIS GROSS
Alpha Beta® Daily Peel
(Universal or Extra Strength)

Should we just deal with the elephant in the room? This is expensive. Not 'remortgage-your-house' expensive, but still 'physical-pain-while-handing-over-my-card' expensive. I don't normally recommend beauty products with prohibitive price points because why start a skincare routine you can't afford to keep up? For this price, I'd expect a product to sing, dance and take my children to school. But in this case, it is worth it. You can expect smoother, brighter, amazing-looking skin, more so the longer you use it. There's a powerful cocktail of exfoliating ingredients that deal with a plethora of issues – hyperpigmentation, dull skin, breakouts, uneven skin texture, overproduction of oil; all pretty impressive. Dr Dennis Gross developed the formulation after using it on the clients at his NYC practice, and you would be hard-pressed to find over-the-counter products that provide the same results. It is quite strong, but not so potent that your face feels raw.

If your skin is sensitive, I'd suggest trying the Universal formula first, and even if you think your face is made of steel, it is still worth doing a patch test (behind your ear) to double check you won't have a reaction.

Still, I hear you ask, 'Is it really worth it?' Well, consider three things. The cost per use is cheaper than an expensive but mediocre facial but yields better results. It is easy to use and easy to travel with. And a friend who has used it from the outset now has such flawless skin you would need a magnifying glass to find her pores. Is that the kind of skin you want? I rest my case.

THE INKEY LIST™
Lactic Acid

I LOVE The Inkey List. The biggest selling point is that the brand is making skincare accessible for everyone, and that accessibility is not just about the very reasonable prices. So many brands have product descriptions so academic you have no idea what they are, or what they do, but The Inkey List is refreshingly straight talking. There are a few products I like in their range, but I have chosen the Lactic Acid to feature here because it is the one that really targets issues of hyperpigmentation (one of the biggest concerns for those with darker skin tones) but does it in a way that is genial and moisturising, as opposed to harsh and stripping. If you are new to acids, this is good entry-level stuff. On opening the bottle, the clear liquid is bubble-bath foamy, which is slightly disconcerting. Thankfully, when it goes onto the skin, there is nothing remotely soapy about it. It is like a very light serum that sinks in beautifully but leaves a matte, yet moisturised, finish. I asked my husband to have a sniff, and he shrugged and said, 'It just smells like a chemical.' He's not wrong (it has 'acid' in the name, so you can't expect it to smell like morello cherries), but don't let that scare you. This is one of the good guys. As it is wallet friendly, it is constantly sold out; so if you do come across it in stock, don't dither, just buy it.

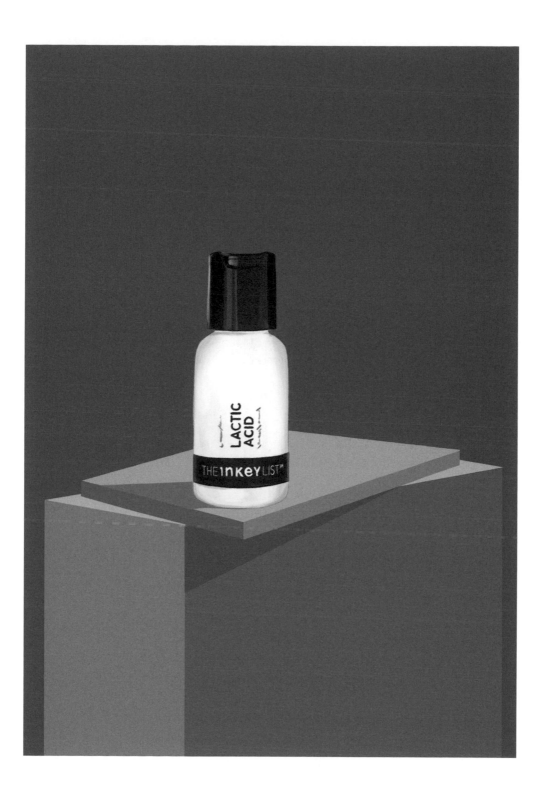

SUNDAY RILEY
Good Genes Glycolic Acid Treatment

Good Genes had long been a cult product when the powers-that-be suddenly realised the lactic-acid content of the exfoliator – a decongesting, smoothing, hyperpigmentation-busting wonder – didn't meet EU regulations, and so Good Genes had to be pulled from every UK retailer for reformulation. Skincare fanatics went into meltdown. Rumours of black-market-style dealings were rife. There was a plethora of die hard fans that couldn't care less that it was now illegal; damn the consequences, they were willing to exchange money under the counter to get their glow fix.

Sunday Riley reformulated and came back a few months later. It has now been renamed Good Genes Glycolic Acid Treatment because the lactic-acid content has been reduced, and glycolic is now the star. People generally don't like change, and I'm sure if you found a box of the original lurking somewhere, you could sell the batch to an addict for the price of a second-hand car. But you know what? I prefer the new one. It is beautifully silky, and it disappears effortlessly into the skin. The change in acids used hasn't affected the results negatively at all. Glycolic has smaller molecules, so it penetrates deeper into the skin and acts like a colonic for your pores. Dead, sun-damaged and speckled skin is still sloughed off and repaired. And you still see a difference after just one use. Again, this might not be so great for sensitive-skin types. While the ingredients include fermented prickly pear to reduce the potential for irritation, the fact is lactic acid is gentler than glycolic. So, sensitive skins, don't be like people who just because they eat a half-decent salad for once in their lives suddenly claim to be a vegan; take your time, suss it out and then see how you go before committing. For those with more robust skin, the new incarnation of Good Genes is a very good thing indeed.

THIS WORKS®
Evening Detox Spray-On Exfoliant

This really works! Where do I even begin? My addiction to this product knows no bounds. This is the spray-on exfoliant that gives me such glossy, light-reflecting skin that even the most highly polished wood floor would have trouble competing. I can honestly say the results are akin to that of a brilliant facial. I'm also impressed by the packaging – I am slightly cack-handed with liquid exfoliators so the spray format is a dream (why hasn't anybody thought of it sooner?). Key ingredients are salicylic acid (to tackle congestion, blemishes, breakouts and even fine lines), witch hazel (antibacterial and anti-inflammatory, brilliant for oily skin), and a blend of antioxidants that fight free radicals and the effects of pollution. They advise to use at night, but I spray it on in the morning after washing my face, I spray it on at night after washing my face, I spray it on again while I'm sitting on the sofa watching Netflix, and I spray it on again when I go up to bed. I am addicted.

BIOLOGIQUE RECHERCHE
Lotion P50 PIGM 400

What makes this particular liquid exfoliant above and beyond, is that it was created specifically to deal with hyperpigmentation. It has an unusual dual-acting formulation made up of active ingredients – such as wakame, seaweed and watercress sprout – that not only reduce the intensity of dark spots that already exist but prevent new ones from forming. Of course, like all Biologique Recherche products, it doesn't smell great. Have you ever boiled fresh snapper scales in a big pan of water? No? Neither have I. But let's just imagine for a moment. After sifting it through a sieve, what do you end up with? A clear broth with a hint of fish. That is what this smells like. Faint, but it's there. It is slightly disorientating, and I can't focus on anything else until I wash it off my hands, by which point the scent disappears and I get on with the rest of my day. Why, I hear you ask, do you keep using it? Because this damn thing works. I do it so I don't have to look in the mirror every day and see speckles of dark spots and patches of uneven skin. I am all in, and you will be too.

ALPHA-H
Liquid Gold™

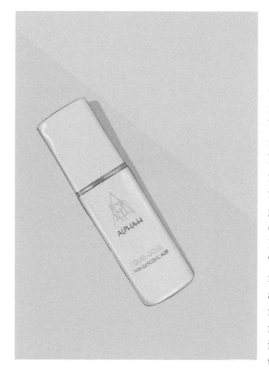

In beauty product terms, this feels like a first-born child. When you are juggling so many products, all vying for your attention, the ones that were there right at the beginning invariably get forgotten. I want to make amends and give credit where it is due. Liquid Gold was the first liquid exfoliator I ever discovered. Except, back then, I had no idea what on earth it was. No one did. The category for liquid exfoliator did not exist; the term had not been coined. I remember being unsure of how and when to use it. After cleansing? Before moisturising? Do I rinse it off? Will I go blind if it gets in my eye? Can I use it in the morning and night without my face feeling like it's on fire? The only thing I knew – from the smug early adopters in Australia, from where this brand derives – is that it gives you implausibly lovely skin. And so, of course, I wanted a piece of the pie. Once I began to use it, I learnt a few things. It's a 'peel while you sleep' situation. This sounds much scarier than it is, but just think of it as an overnight treatment that you don't need to rinse off. It stimulates skin-cell renewal, so you swiftly notice a difference in your skin texture. It penetrates deep into the pores and targets bacteria, making it a go-to for anyone suffering from breakouts and acne. One of the key ingredients is liquorice – an unsung hero that is so amazing for treating hyperpigmentation, I'm amazed more brands don't include it in their formulations. You start out using it every other night so your skin can build up resistance, but sensitive skin types should bypass completely – this is too harsh for you (sorry!). For everyone else, it's genius.

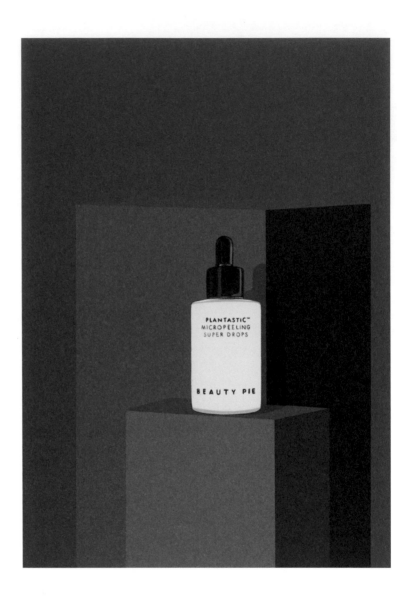

BEAUTY PIE™
Plantastic™ Micropeeling Super Drops

Not all cults are bad. Case in point: Beauty Pie and its ardent followers. Of which I am one. These drops are one of my many favourites in the range. For any skincare newbies, the word 'micropeeling' probably sounds alarming, but it's really not. It should not be confused with 'microneedling', which is essentially puncturing the skin with teeny needles in order to stimulate the production of collagen (it's what keeps the tone and firmness of skin). Microneedling I would advise only having done by an expert on darker skin tones, otherwise you will leave – with a face worse than you started with – in a taxi for fear of scaring the general public. I speak from experience.

These drops, on the other hand, are a breeze. Most liquid exfoliators have a watery texture, a chemical scent and a tingle that we accept, because that's what you expect from something that nibbles away at your dead skin. This clever product, however, bucks the trend. It is plant based – so incredibly gentle – and has the consistency of a luxe serum. The blurb on the website describes it as a '24/7 glow-giving one-serum wonder'. It is right. This really is a powerful skin transformer, without the bravado of many of its counterparts. I find that when I use this – a few drops are all you need – I am less susceptible to breakouts; my skin is much more hydrated and significantly more even toned. I didn't see these results overnight, so if you are expecting to douse this on and wake up with a new face, don't. Where this product scores, however, is that it is gentle enough to be used daily and so the journey to great skin feels less brutal. Additionally, it is suitable for every skin type. The price you pay for the quality makes this a steal, and unless you are drinking the stuff, it will last you ages. I'm a believer.

NEOGEN DERMALOGY
Bio-Peel⁺ Gauze Peeling Wine Pads

Thirty exfoliating pads soaked in wine. Not the drinking kind, mind you, but rather the kind that revolutionises your skin. If you expect to dip your face in Merlot and get the same results, you'll be disappointed. The star ingredient is resveratrol, an antioxidant derivative of red wine, which has naturally occurring AHAs to slough off dead skin cells, protect your skin from pigmentation and premature ageing, declog your pores and, bottom line, give you a brighter complexion. I mean, if you asked for more, it would just be greedy. The texture of the pads is interesting. Smooth one side, slightly rough on the other; it works both for those who love physical exfoliation, as well as those who prefer a chemical to do the work. And then there's the wine-red colour. Call it out of step with an industry currently obsessed with everything 'natural', but I am totally into it. Plus, the smell! Nostalgically sweet, fruity and juicy, it reminds me of the bubblegum my sister and I used to steal from our grandmother's convenience store on the outskirts of Lagos. I love the fact that the pads have a big surface area, making them easier to use. Most exfoliating pads on the market are so small that using them feels akin to stepping out of the bath and trying to dry yourself with a handkerchief. If I had a teeny complaint, it would be that the pads are perhaps soaked a little too generously and the product ends up dripping everywhere. But it gives me glass skin (Google it), so I'll stop moaning.

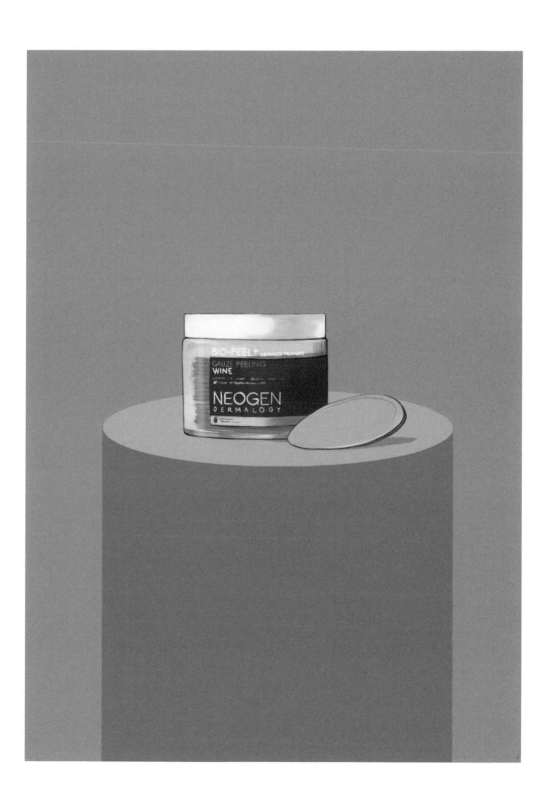

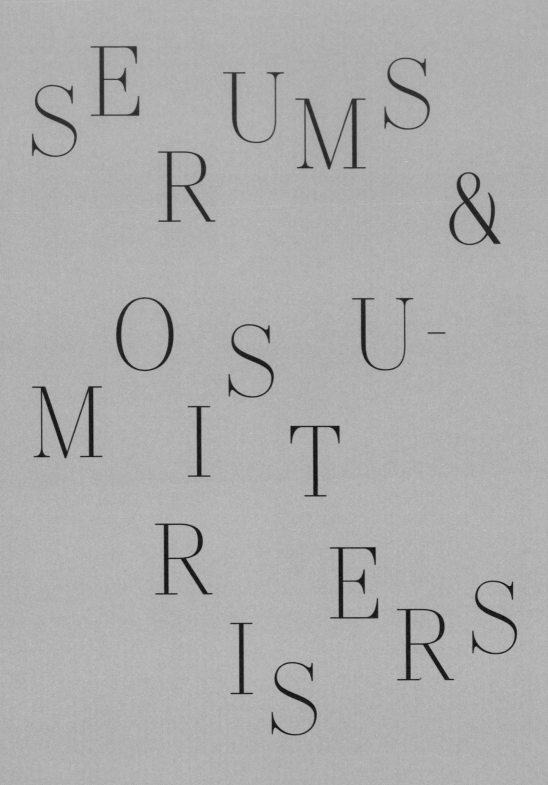

SERUMS & MOISTURISERS

THINGS TO NOTE...

Think of moisturisers like winter
clothes: the better you layer, the more
effective they are. There are three key
ingredients in any grown-up skincare
routine: retinol (just don't mainline
it); hyaluronic acid (to keep your face
plump and fresh) and vitamin C (to
ensure you no longer look as though a
grey cloud has just landed on your face).

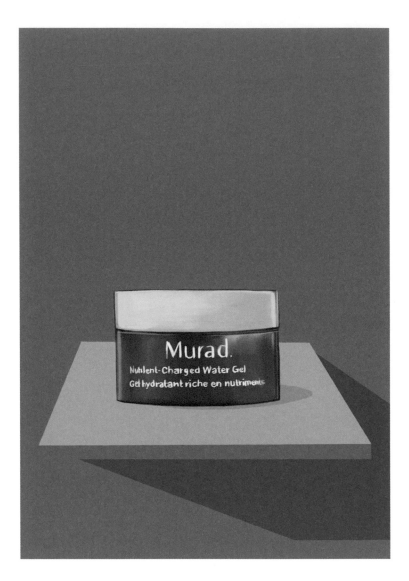

MURAD®
Nutrient-Charged
Water Gel

Once upon a time, before my beauty editor days, I was terrified of moisturisers. I think people who live with the saga of oily skin generally are. For me, 'moisturisers' were a euphemism for 'I'm coming to clog your pores!'. So, after a lifetime of choosing what I now realise were simply inappropriate moisturisers, I decided to skip the process entirely. (Extreme, I know. A bit like joining the convent just because you've had a few rubbish relationships.) I began to stick to 'treatment' products – to combat acne, blemishes and oily skin – and leave it at that. This, of course, was problematic: many of these treatments were stripping, meaning moisturising should really have been a crucial aspect of my regime. I'd end up with a face so Spandex tight and itchy, my smile couldn't hide the fact I was actually wincing in discomfort. To make matters worse, the oiliness once limited to my T-zone suddenly became more pervasive. Thank God for a facialist I met years ago. Through her, I learnt that it is possible to have skin that is both oily and dehydrated and, by stripping it, your skin will compensate by producing more oil and continue to be dehydrated ... it becomes this catch-22 situation. My oily skin essentially needed hydration, and there is a way to do this without adding pore blockers to your regime. And here is where this pretty pink, slightly rose-scented water gel excels. My skin drinks up the concoction of vitamins, peptides and minerals like the gluttonous protagonist of *The Tiger Who Came to Tea*. The lightweight texture is perfect in warm weather – and under foundation – but I use it year-round. It doesn't do anything fancy like blitzing acne, blemishes, pigmentation and so forth, but if you are in the market for a great oil-free, skin-plumping moisturiser, then this is it.

INDEED LABS™
Boosters

If you were to take a picture of my ever-expanding skincare collection, the first thing you would notice is the ridiculous number of little bottles, usually no more than 30ml, with a squeezy rubber thing on top. The proper name for them is a pipette (also referred to as droppers) and they help to dispense the correct amount of product, so you don't use more than you need. This is great for people like me, who would otherwise drown their faces with serum – more is more is more, and all that. Six of my favourite serums come under the Indeed Laboratories umbrella. When these launched into the market and were touted as 'boosters', I thought they might be yet another baffling skincare category we'd just have to get our heads around. However, it really isn't that complicated. Think of boosters like your spice and seasoning cupboard. What you use is down to the individual. Some people think it's OK to season chicken with nothing but its own juices (good luck with that – please don't invite me to dinner), while others might want to use a combination of onions, thyme, rosemary, black pepper and so on. Boosters are like that, adding as much or as little flavour as you want. If you get the combination right for your skin's needs,

the results are fabulous. They can be mixed into your existing skincare products but are just as effective when used alone. The one thing they have in common is that they are all quite light, meaning they sink gloriously into the skin and leave a lovely glow. They also layer beautifully, meaning they don't pill when you add something else on top.

The **Q10**, says the brand, is anti-ageing, a term I neither like nor relate to. I mean, yes, no one aspires to be a prune, but it would be nice if brands could use more positive terminology. All anti-ageing does is fuel a ridiculous pursuit of a youthfulness that is unrealistic and unattainable. Ageing is not the most terrible thing that could happen to a woman: after all, if you didn't age, you'd be dead. Anyway, anti-ageing aside, it's one of my favourite boosters. The combination of coenzyme Q10 and vitamins E and C helps to inhibit the production of pigment, even out skin tone and minimise fine lines. **Collagen** is all about tightening and toning the skin. I would not automatically tell women of colour to make a beeline for this, because these are not issues I find come up regularly; however, if you find your skin has lost elasticity or volume and just needs a little bit of oomph, give this a shot. **Radiance** and **Hydration** are both exactly what they say on the tin. Radiance makes my skin looks dewy, brighter and, dare I say it, more youthful when I use it. Hydration not only plumps up the skin but also has the added bonus of including niacinamide, which regulates sebum production and improves congestion. I love this ingredient – especially now I can pronounce it without sounding illiterate. It's easy when you split it into three words: Nia. Cina. Mide; the last word rhymes with 'died' as opposed to 'bidet'. **Resistance** boosts your skin's capacity to resist damage (pollution and UV), combats pigmentation and minimises breakouts. Stressed-out skin will love the **Mineral** booster, which detoxifies, improves the circulation of oxygen to the skin and protects the skin from glycation – that's the premature ageing that begins to show up on your skin when you have too much sugar in your bloodstream. Yes, people, this is for real: the less sugar you eat, the better your skin looks. I know. I'm sorry.

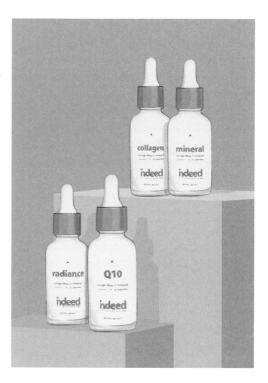

VICHY
Normaderm Phytosolution Double-Correction Daily Care Moisturiser

As a teen battling acne, it felt like every skincare product available either stripped my skin or clogged it up. What I didn't realise then – and it is still news to many today – is that every skin, regardless of its condition, needs hydrating. Yes, even the oily, pimple-ridden ones like mine was at the time. But how does one hydrate problematic skin while simultaneously treating it? Well, this moisturiser, created to target blemishes and breakouts, might just have the answer. Its formula is a clever combination of exfoliating salicylic acid and hydrating hyaluronic acid, which delivers on its promise that you will see clearer skin within a week. How my 14-year-old self would have loved it. While I am no longer an acne sufferer, like so many adults these days I still find myself battling the occasional breakout (apparently modern-day stress levels have driven our cortisone levels through the roof, meaning that adult breakouts and acne are on the rise – thank you, life). With its pore-friendly, water-light texture, this easily sinks into skin, acting quickly to restore balance and leaving a radiant finish and pleasantly cooling feeling. It has a slight, fleeting menthol scent, but truth be told, I'm so impressed with this moisturiser, I wouldn't care if it smelt like Deep Heat.

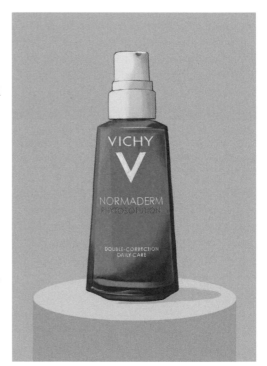

DRUNK ELEPHANT
Lala Retro™
Whipped Cream

As a fan of gossamer-thin moisturisers, I normally run a mile from creamy formulas. This, however, is an exception. Don't be put off by the 'cream' in the name: in reality, this is soufflé-light and nourishes skin without asphyxiating it. The fragrance-free formula combines six African oils, including baobab and marula, to moisturise and defend the skin, vitamin C and plantain extract for their brightening properties, and fermented green tea to help combat fine lines. If you are using a lot of acids in your skincare regime, this works well to soothe your skin and give it a much-needed hydration injection. Sensitive skins will also be pleased to know this has a perfect PH level, so your skin won't be thrown off kilter. If your skin is very dry, however, you may find it guzzles this down greedily whilst demanding more, so do consider an extra layer of something richer. If your skin is oily then, yes, you can use it too – it won't clog your pores – but unless you have a gold-standard, workaholic make-up primer, I'd save this for bedtime.

SHISEIDO
Ultimune Power Infusing Concentrate

Have you seen *Dynasty*? No, not the new one; the original big-in-the-80s soap, where all the women had poofy hair, too much make-up, shoulder pads and glittery frocks. It was hyperbolic to an almost pantomime degree, and it made for fabulous viewing. When I look at this serum, I think of *Dynasty*. It could have quite easily had a part in the show. The packaging – Glossy! Red! Gold! – is so of that era and the complete antithesis of the minimalist, pared-down, Instagrammable beauty products that are so ubiquitous right now. But that's where the nostalgia stops. As with most Japanese beauty brands, the actual product formulation is seriously advanced – and it is utterly brilliant. A concoction of reishi mushroom, iris root, gingko, Japanese shiso and thyme strengthens the skin, making it able to resist the damage that comes from environmental factors, such as pollution and stress, while also shielding the skin from premature ageing. It works, and so I love this thin white liquid, which looks like palm wine but smells like an old-fashioned face powder. I tend to layer it with other really thin serums, but even on its own I find it leaves my skin smoother, super hydrated, much more supple and plumper (the stats from all the women they trialled with this product also attest to this). Still, there is no getting away from the fact that this one is quite expensive, and it doesn't last ages. But I will say this: when I don't use this serum, no one tells me how great my skin looks. What they do say is, 'You look like you need a break.' When I do use this serum, my skin looks healthier and completely hides the fact that I spend half my life (and probably my income) drinking gallons of extra-hot cappuccino.

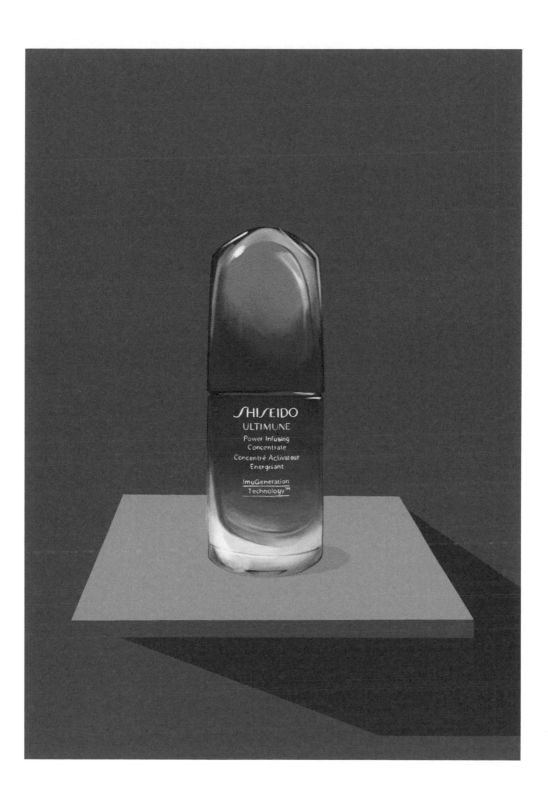

PAULA'S CHOICE
Nightly Reconditioning Moisturizer

As much as I champion Paula's Choice, this is the first moisturiser from the brand with which I have truly fallen in love. It is designed to work overnight to neutralise any environmental aggressors with which you may have come into contact during the day – such as pollution and blue light from your devices – while also prepping your skin so it is ready to fight any pollution the next day. There is evidence to show that these environmental aggressors have a negative impact on the quality of our skin so, at the risk of sounding preachy, it is probably worth paying attention. The key superfood/antioxidant ingredients here include wild cherry, flaxseed and arugula; they have been scientifically proven to strengthen the skin's barrier. If you have severely dehydrated skin, however, I think you'll need to apply an extra layer of something super hydrating – a good hyaluronic acid perhaps – as the finish is matte. I prefer dewiness but as I only use it at night, and it feels comfortable on the skin, the finish isn't relevant. The key for me is how my skin looks and feels when I wake up in the morning, and with this it is smoother, even, and with no greasy patches. By the way, those patches of oil that make you want to rush to wash your face are a sign that whatever you have used has upset your PH balance, and your skin is freaked out. The texture of this one, a gel–lotion hybrid, is a little thicker than I'd normally go for, but to its credit it doesn't feel heavy on the skin. The scent isn't bad – a nutty cherry – but those with an aversion to anything scented or gourmand inspired might take issue with it. I'd wager that once you think of the upsides – a skin-balancing moisturiser that prevents the light emitting from your (cracked) iPhone from destroying your face – the scent won't be a big deal.

KIEHL'S
Ultra Facial Moisturizer

We've become so consumed by the nascent skin hydration product categories that we've somewhat cast away the merits of the humble moisturiser – a bit like the man who trades the wife of his youth for a much younger model. Sure, the moisturiser is old school – she was courting the beauty consumer long before serums became the star of the R&D lab – but that doesn't make her any less relevant. Find the right one for you and she will hydrate your skin and help it retain its moisture without leaving it feeling greasy. This skin-softening offering by Kiehl's is such a moisturiser: creamy but light, and beautifully absorbent. The anti-fragrance brigade will also be glad to hear the scent is non-descript (I see your victorious air punch). Key ingredients include squalane,

a brilliant hydrating oil; vitamin A, a very gentle retinol to slow down signs of ageing; and vitamin E to protect the skin from environmental stressors. I personally love the formula, however it would be disingenuous of me to say it works for everyone. Thankfully, Kiehl's has something for all skin types: oily skins who may find this a little too heavy can turn to the **Ultra Facial Oil Free Gel Cream**. Skins which are older or incredibly dry are best suited to the heavier cream version, **Ultra Facial Cream**. But for anyone with 'normal', sensitive and combination skins, the Ultra Facial Moisturizer is a dream. It might not be fancy or new, but just remember: newness doesn't always mean best.

SARAH CHAPMAN
Skinesis Overnight Facial

I am on the fence when it comes to facial oils. My cynical blanket statement is that I think many people like to use them for their sensorial aspect, not their results. It's easy to convince yourself that an unctuous-textured product is improving the quality of your skin when, in fact, many facial oils on the market still haven't nailed the efficacy of their formulations. Sarah Chapman, on the other hand, has. Chapman, the brilliant facialist behind Meghan Markle's flawless complexion, knows a thing or two about skin (a Sarah Chapman facial is a sublime experience), so it isn't surprising that this formulation is superb. Don't be fooled by the packaging: you don't get very much in the bottle, and its opaque nature means you never know when it's close to being emptied (frustrating), but park that thought and consider instead that it's a night-time routine game changer. Beautifully scented – jasmine, rose, tuberose and frangipani – this oil is a blend of protective antioxidants, vitamins A and C to smooth, plump and brighten the skin, and advanced technologies to boost collagen and increase skin cells' life span. It is not greasy so you won't wake up with clogged pores and stained bed linen. Instead, you will look like you've had a facial – overnight.

SKINCEUTICALS
C E Ferulic

If you tried a quick sample of this, you might ask yourself, why on earth should I pay this much money for something that smells like hot-dog water? And yet, in spite of the unappealing scent and frankly astronomical price, it is SkinCeuticals' best-selling product. Why? Because you'll be hard-pressed to find anything that does what this does. 'Never mind what it does, what on earth is it?' was my question when I was initially introduced to it years ago. As I share the key points
I learnt, just pretend you're back in school and try to concentrate. It is a highly potent antioxidant serum that enhances your protection against environmental damage – especially when used with sunscreen. Ferulic acid (found in the cell walls of plants) is high in the antioxidant that reverses and prevents photo damage. The C in the name stands for vitamin C; the E, vitamin E. They all work in synergy to improve the appearance of lines, wrinkles and hyperpigmentation – think of them like the ultimate 'choir' to make your skin sing. What makes C E Ferulic special (and expensive) is this: the serum incorporates the purest and highest concentration of vitamin C, which is amalgamated with Ferulic acid and vitamin E in a way that is stable, which means the formulation doesn't fall apart and stop working. Apparently, this is impossible without an Einstein level of cold-hearted science, hence why the formulation is patented, and the beauty cognoscenti are obsessed. Phew.

The following points are more important to keep in mind. It is a lightweight oil-meets-water liquid that should be applied every morning. Keep it airtight in a cool area away from direct sunlight – the fridge is good – so it doesn't lose its potency. Follow it with your moisturiser and make sure you also use it on your neck and décolletage (that's the no man's land between your neck and the top of your chest). Skip the latter step and after a while you'll notice your face looks stunningly youthful while the rest of you looks borrowed from a long dead ancestor. The serum is incredibly concentrated, so you only need a few drops, which is just as well, considering how expensive it is. Anyone suffering from acne scarring and breakouts will find this to be an extraordinary friend, and everyone can expect the kind of skin that will make them never want to wear foundation again: it's that magnificent.

FRESH
Rose Deep Hydration Face Cream

The 'rose' on this product's name is quite literal. It has been created with both rosewater and pure rose flower oil, so it does actually smell like a bunch of roses, albeit the expensive ones you buy from a chic elevated florist rather than the wilted version from your local petrol station. If you find rose scents unbearable, I doubt anything I say from here on will convince you to tap into this product. Everyone else, read on. Don't be fooled by the 'cream' element in the title: the texture is cream-like but not dense in the way we have all come to expect. Rather it looks like a fat-free yogurt, which means it absorbs easily and quickly rather than just sitting on your skin like a procrastinator with a deadline. Along with the aforementioned rose elements and vitamin E – all known for their soothing and nourishing properties – it is brimming with hyaluronic acid, angelica leaf, which helps the retention of moisture, and a time-release technology that keeps skin hydrated over 24 hours, elevating it far beyond your bog-standard moisturiser. Normal-to-dry skins can expect plump, soft and wonderfully hydrated skin as a result, although if your skin is oily this will be a disaster under your make-up, so save it for night-time. My little quibble is that whilst aesthetically, I love the glass jar, for practical and hygiene purposes I think a tube would fare much better. Nevertheless, it is a brilliant, sensorial moisturiser which does everything it says on the pot. As long as you love roses, you'll love it.

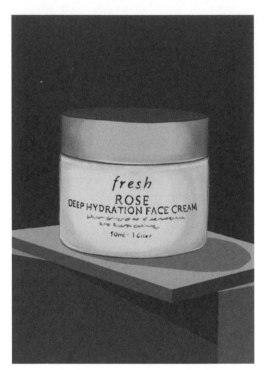

ZELENS
Z Luminous Brightening Serum

I was having a conversation recently with a fellow journalist as to how much is too much to pay for a beauty product. Some people are addicted to super expensive products, which, they claim, have transformed their skin. I, on the other hand, swear most of these are placebos. I really believe that with technology and formulations being so advanced it is possible to find less expensive alternatives that are totally on a par with the more expensive stuff. I also believe there are some exceptions. For me, this pigmentation-busting brightening serum is one. Yes, it does have a hefty price tag. Yes, there's only 30ml in a bottle. And, yes, I am in bewilderment looking at my own half-empty bottle and wondering how the hell that went down so quickly. But then I look in the mirror, and I have all the justification I need. It is utterly incredible and above and beyond the numerous brightening serums I've used. So many 'brightening serums' don't actually brighten whereas, with this, I began to see a difference in my skin pretty much straight away. The formulation is superior, unsurprisingly, because the founder, Dr Marko Lens, is a world-renowned skincare expert. The cocktail of radiance-boosting ingredients includes niacinamide (which helps to reduce dark spots, even skin tone and increase the skin's elasticity), resorcinol (regulates melanin production), phytic acid (exfoliates) and hyaluronic acid (boosts moisture levels). The dreamy texture is also worth a mention; beautifully light and exquisite-smelling. The one thing that really sets this serum apart from its rivals is that it gives you such an epic, addictive glow that I call 'luminosity on speed'. Like me, you will be tempted to slather on tons of it, but I'm learning you don't actually need very much, so resist and just use one-two drops max (I probably don't need to tell you that – the price tag is quite enough to motivate frugality).

The directions say follow it with a moisturiser – not necessary for oilier skin types; however, if you feel it is necessary, go for something super light, like a pure hyaluronic acid. The non-negotiable is suncare. Unless you want your pigmentation issues to be like annoying family members who come to visit and never leave, applying SPF is not a step I recommend you skip.

VICHY
Minéral 89 Serum

I am constantly working on dismantling my prejudices about certain 'genres' or trends in beauty. For example, when it comes to anything to do with crystals, I cannot roll my eyes enough. If someone waxes lyrical about 'this really great brand', my ears prick up. Once they add 'and they use the healing power of rose quartz' my brain immediately starts mulling over more exciting things, like which brand of dishwasher tablets I need to buy on my way home. Mass-market skincare brands are also a genre with which I have had an issue in the past. I have no issue with inexpensive products, but like everyone else, ultimately, I want stuff that works and doesn't bring me out in hives. My problem with the mass-market beauty world is that I never felt that I, a person of colour with skincare issues that are particular to the melanin in my skin, am on their radar.

But the efficacy of this Vichy product changed that. It is like a huge glass of water for the skin. I'll be honest, drinking water does not fill me with excitement. One of my pet hates is hearing supermodels say their beauty secret is 'drinking lots of water'. But as clichéd and boring as it is, drinking water does make a huge difference to the skin. Give up coffee for a month and up your intake of water, and you'll see. Yes, you'll probably have lost all your friends due to your extreme grumpiness from the withdrawal symptoms, but you will have better skin. If that's too extreme, this serum is the next best thing (well, sort of). It is fortified with hyaluronic acid and a blend of minerals that hydrates and plumps up the skin while also protecting it from pollution and other environmental aggressors. I love the superlight watery-gel texture (it is deeply hydrating but non-greasy), and it is oil free, which for someone with oily skin is the dream. If you have dry and/or dehydrated skin – be it from the use of peels, exfoliators or a pitiful lack of water intake – then you also need this thirst-quencher. If you have sensitive skin, this is cooling and calming, and will not irritate your skin. The best thing about this, however, is that it does wonders for my productivity. I keep it by my desk when I am writing from home. When I get writer's block, I take a moment to slather on another layer. It's a great distraction from getting up for the hundredth time to see what else is left in the fridge to eat.

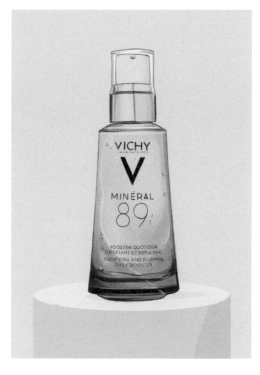

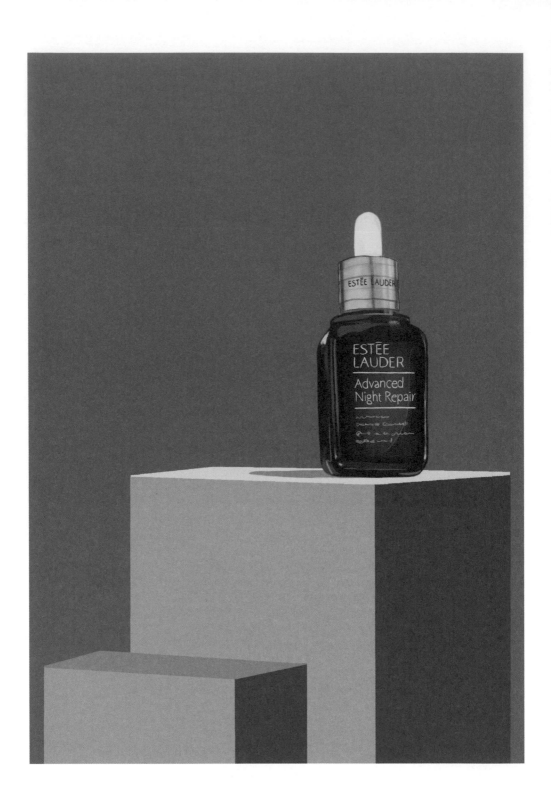

ESTĒE LAUDER
Advanced Night Repair Synchronized Recovery Complex II

Whenever I get up in the middle of the night to go to the loo, I cannot resist looking in the mirror (albeit briefly) before heading back to bed. Why do I do it? Not because I have narcissistic tendencies that rage unrestrained even when I'm desperate to empty my bladder. It's because I've discovered that what my skin looks like at that point in the night is a great indicator as to how well (or not) my night-time skincare is working. I've had some nights of trying new products, and during the loo run I'll notice my face just lacks a certain freshness. This manifests in a number of ways: patches of greasiness loitering on my forehead, uneven skin tone, pores that look deeper than a gully. And just... grubby. While I will concede that there are tons of things that affect the condition of your skin at night – insomnia, hormones, stress and so on – you just know when it's not working. I feel we have the tendency to keep going with products that are not producing results just because other people have said how great they are. Remember, it's all very personal. We need to start treating our beauty products like famous people treat their romantic relationships: if they're not working, get rid and replace. Advanced Night Repair

(ANR for short) is the replacement that always passes the loo-run test. It's 40 years old but has recently been ever so slightly reformulated, so the new blurb now says that it is suitable for every ethnicity. This might seem like a tiny, irrelevant detail, but I think it is significant in the move for brands to be more inclusive. Beauty brands, take note. I had friends in the industry who were obsessed with this serum, but I didn't necessarily think it was speaking to me. However, at the end of the day, I'm a beauty editor, and I needed to know what the fuss was about. Well, it is totally worth the hype. The effect on the skin is striking. This is down to the cocktail of antioxidants, hyaluronic acid and, most especially, a patented clock gene technology in the serum. The critical repairing process of our skin declines as we age; this technology helps skin to renew itself more quickly and at the right time every night. I know it says night repair, but I like to live on the edge, so I also use it during the day. So many serums make your foundation slide around, but this sits really well under make-up, enhancing it even – mixing it with foundation and a liquid highlighter gives you a really elevated finish. It has been a best-seller for years, and I see why – especially on my 2am loo run.

THE ORDINARY
"Buffet" / Niacinamide 10% + Zinc 1%

The Ordinary's website is terrifying. I often advise people to head to The Ordinary to get their skincare fix because it is the one place where they will get exactly what they need and be able to afford to keep on using it. Everyone, initially, comes back dazed, panic-stricken and empty-handed. I understand.

The Ordinary pioneered hi–lo beauty and add that to the chic black-and-white minimalist finish, and you have a winning situation. It is the most utterly brilliant, democratic skincare brand. No question. The issue is understanding; it's exhausting to establish what everything does, how you use it, when you use it. No one wants to lose the will to live over a moisturiser. So, with that in mind, I'll cut through the noise and tell you about my two mainstays. **"Buffet"** is a relatively easy one to decipher. Have you ever been to an all-you-can-eat in the States? This is the skincare version – the ultimate feast for your skin. It has a bunch of skin-loving, 'anti-ageing' ingredients (numerous amino acids, peptides, hyaluronic acid). I use a couple of drops after my liquid exfoliator, and because it isn't sticky or tacky, it layers well. This is super important – I can't stand it when you layer on a serum, and it starts to bobble like an old jumper. The **Niacinamide 10% + Zinc 1%** is another key part of my skincare regime, and if you are a member of the blemish-battling oily-skin crew, then this is essential. It targets congestion, evens out the skin tone and regulates sebum production. It also improves moisture retention, which means your skin never feels stripped. Remember, it is not a moisturiser, so I would layer something extra on top, nothing too heavy (something like **Murad's Nutrient-Charged Water Gel** and **NIOD's Multi-Molecular Hyaluronic Complex** would work well). Unsurprisingly, the product is a best-seller and frequently out of stock; if you find some, stock-pile. So, there you go: a quick lesson on The Ordinary skincare range. Well, not quite, but it is enough to keep you going while you get the degree needed to help you decipher the rest.

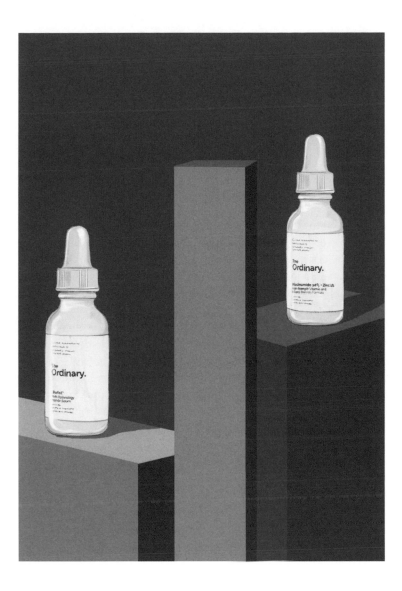

MARKS AND SPENCER
Formula Absolute
Ultimate Sleep Cream

Everyone is tired, but unlike being 'busy', no one goes around boasting about it because there's no glory in it. Which is good because this night cream won't make you less busy but it will make you look less tired. Research proves that sleep and your nightly regime (or lack of the above) has a direct effect on the complex cell renewal process that happens overnight. Which is why you need something that does an epic job of working that night shift. The tagline for this cream is 'Skin that makes you look like you've had 8 hours' sleep' and when it launched in 2016, it sold out and created a frenzied waiting list. Believe the hype. The texture alone is worthy of praise: unlike most night creams, which lean towards the thick and heavy, this is rich but lightweight and unlikely to result in breakouts. 71 per cent of women who trialled it said it transformed their skin in two weeks. I have no idea how many of those were of darker skin tones but I will say this: I first used it as an exhausted semi-human on an overnight flight and my skin did, as a result, look less fatigued, brighter (a key ingredient is the dark-spot reducer niacinamide) and hydrated (thank you plumping hyaluronic acid). I wouldn't generally suggest this for oily skins – drier, more mature skins would fare better here – however for arid conditions, it's worth considering. All this shows that expensive night creams aren't always the best. This one, a low-priced contingency found in middle England's favourite store famed for its food and lingerie blows its pricey peers out of the water.

SUNDAY RILEY
Tidal Brightening Enzyme Water Cream

One day I met up with an old acquaintance, a beauty obsessive in the wrong job, whom I hadn't seen for years. We trash-talked bad beauty products on the market (there are a lot of those around) and gushed over their superior counterparts. It was all very earnest; you'd think we were discussing world issues as opposed to the joys of a moisturiser that stops you shedding like a snake. And then she asked me what I thought of Tidal, and I confessed I had never used it. Her intake of breath was so severe, the look of mortification on her face so intense, I thought she was going to pass out. I'm convinced I went so far down in her estimation that come to think of it, I haven't actually heard from her since. So, of course, I had to try this. And Oh. My. Goodness. It is sublime. The name suggests this eau-de-nil-coloured marvel is a cream, but it is not actually creamy per se. It is the texture of a barely there, no-sugar no-fat no-nothing-added yogurt. Shocking for your tastebuds, delicious for your skin.

The main ingredients make a stellar cast: hyaluronic acid and tamarind to plump up and eradicate fine lines, alpha-arbutin to brighten and even skin tone, and papaya enzymes to refine skin texture. It is the one moisturiser with a water-like texture that also exfoliates – the enzymes pull apart all those dead skin cells – and reduces hyperpigmentation. It sinks in beautifully and gives you the glow of your life, and the intensity is more pronounced if you keep it in the fridge (Korean women have beauty fridges in their homes, and they have incredible skin).

So, dear old acquaintance, I hope you are reading this. I'm sorry for being so slow on the uptake; hope you'll agree I have now redeemed myself.

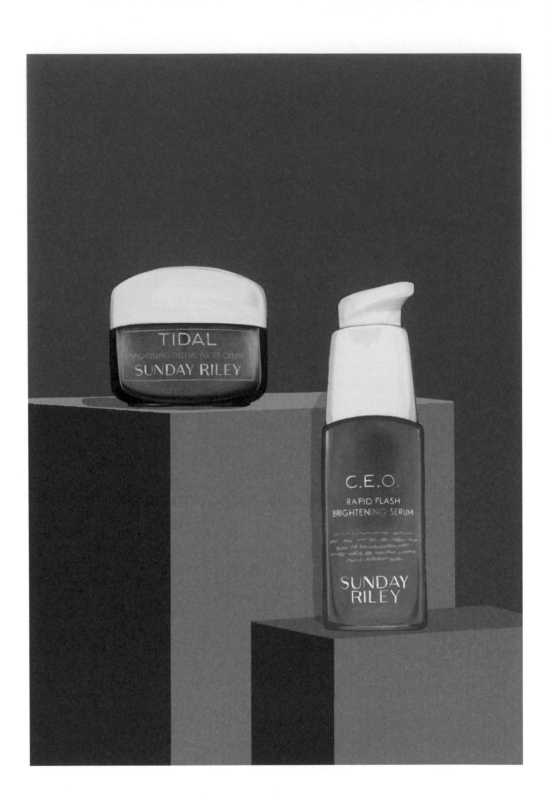

SUNDAY RILEY
C.E.O. Rapid Flash Brightening Serum

There are many things that living in a buzzing city gives you, and one of them is skin that resembles a weary slug crawling off to its deathbed. Of course, if you are one of the world's superhumans, who always has a brilliant skincare regime that never, ever defaults to 'I really cannot be bothered', this will not happen to you. For the rest of humanity, who sometimes take their eye off the ball, at some point bad skin knocks on the door. I started using this serum when I woke up one day and realised my skin looked like an advert for smog. And, goodness, Sunday Riley really didn't come to play with this one. The key word is RAPID. I saw a difference in my skin overnight. Prior to this, I had only used two of Sunday's products: Good Genes, the classic, ingenious exfoliator, and a toner that I banished because the smell was so heinous it threatened to erupt my sinuses. This, on the other hand, is an inoffensive citrus, unless you are one of those strange people who don't like citrus. I have since then immersed myself in the world of Sunday Riley, and I trust the efficacy of the products – Sunday is not just a brand founder, she is also a formulator; so, she knows what she is doing. Still, I was stunned at how quickly and brilliantly this serum delivered its luminosity. It sinks seamlessly into the skin and totally disappears, no pale tinge, no matte, soulless finish. Rather, it is gloriously glossy, and after a little while you start to look as if you have twinkling fairy lights sewn into the fabric of your skin. It also minimises pores, lines and dehydration, and fades acne. The potency is ultimately down to the heavy concentration of vitamin C, an ingredient everyone should have in their beauty arsenal. Do note, however, that there is vitamin C, and there is this stuff, which is gold standard – hence you see the results in a 'flash'.

ELIZABETH ARDEN
Eight Hour® Cream

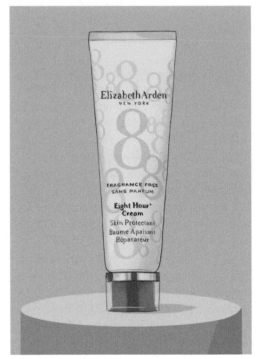

Everyone is obsessed with multitasking.
We'd like to think it's because we are
starved for time but I sometimes wonder if
we just want to prove (read: show off) how
accomplished we are at juggling a million
and one tasks, and debunk the idea that
having it all is not a myth. Alas, there are so
many products on the market now that aim
to be the beauty equivalent of the human
polymath. My experience verifies that most
fail miserably. But then you have the Eight
Hour Cream. There is a good reason why
it has won countless awards: this glossy,
apricot-hued balm – for despite the name,
it has a balmy texture – is a concoction of
vitamin E, salicylic acid and petroleum
(yes, the Vaseline stalwart) that essentially
does everything. If my brows are acting
crazy, this slicks them down. If my skin is
feeling particularly dehydrated or sensitive,
I use it as a night cream. If my cuticles are
dry, it becomes a softener. It is effective
on cuts and grazes, as an eye gloss, post-
sunburn, as a lip balm, as a foot balm...
I could go on. The only thing it doesn't
work on is hands – too sticky. Whilst
I personally love the citronella scent and
feel this is part of its charm, many don't,
but fear not: there is now a fragrance-free
version to keep that contingency of beauty
lovers happy. Either way, once you try it you
won't look back. It is perfection in a tube.

CLINIQUE
Moisture Surge™ Face Spray Thirsty Skin Relief

Some of my greatest beauty discoveries have either happened accidentally or through sheer desperation, such as this spray, which had been a paid-up member of my unopened beauty stash for months, until I had a situation. My overzealous dalliance with dead-skin-shedding acids had left me with a dehydrated and – ironically – dull face, lines I never thought I possessed and a canvas not even the best make-up could look good on. It was a case of too much of a good thing. I needed intense moisture without grease, stickiness or heaviness. The words 'moisture surge' sold this mist to me. Post-cleansing and toning, I spritzed this over my face and, my goodness, the results were astonishing. Like a dead plant in a cartoon, my skin dramatically sprang to life, looking immediately plumper, brighter and dewier. So now, of course, I mainline it. During the day, I layer it between my moisturiser and serum like a hydration sandwich, and in the evening, I repeatedly spritz it in front of the TV. Some people like to use it to prime their skin pre-make-up and set it post-make-up. I wouldn't. Make-up might sit better on hydrated skin, however it's your primer that will stop your make-up shifting around, and your setting spray that will actually 'set' it. This is simply a very good hydrating mist, so use it for what it was created for. I have always been quite cynical about the validity of mists as a beauty category but if they all delivered like the Moisture Surge, the world would be a better place.

Your approa
applying mo
creams shou
clever winter
Numerous th
infinitely mo
than one thi

to
turisers and
emulate
ressing.
layers are
effective
covering.

DRUNK ELEPHANT™
A-Passioni™ Retinol Cream

There are two beauty questions I've been asked by women of all ages, all skin tones and all races. One: Is Drunk Elephant any good? (Do bear in mind that Drunk Elephant is easily, next to Glossier, one of the most hyped launches in the beauty industry for years.) Two: What exactly is retinol?

To answer the first question: yes, Drunk Elephant (DE) is good. Its clever, well-formulated, brilliant products are made without what founder Tiffany Masterson calls 'the suspicious six', i.e. certain ingredients you will find in tons of other beauty products, such as silicones, fragrances and essential oils, which, potentially, can disrupt the skin. This free-from approach ticks a lot of people's conscious-beauty boxes. For those asking about efficacy and whether, due to its high price point (don't be fooled by the colourful packaging, it's expensive) you could get similar results from other products at a lesser price, the answer is yes and no. There are some products that, I believe, are great, but you can get similar results with other products that cost less.

There are however products in the DE range that are in a class of their own, like this retinol cream, which leads me to the second question. Retinol is basically vitamin A. If you are aged 30 upwards (and are not pregnant or an eczema sufferer) retinol should be in your beauty arsenal. It smooths, minimises and prevents wrinkles, exfoliates dull skin, regulates oily skin, stops your pores from getting clogged up and, over time, evens out pigmentation, dark spots and sun spots. You can see why everyone raves about it. Never mind triple threat, this is everything threat. The thing is, retinol has a reputation for irritating the skin – causing dryness and flaking – so you are advised to stagger its use and introduce it into your regime gradually. Unsurprisingly, most people are scared to even go down that route and that is where DE comes in like a fairy godmother. Their retinol offering is different. Yes, you do still have to stagger your use (once a week to start with, until your skin builds up tolerance – most issues of irritation are down to misuse) but, unlike many other retinol products, you can use it morning and night (just don't forget to layer with extra hydration and wear SPF in the day). The cutting-edge creamy concoction has been created to give maximum results and minimal irritation. At 1 per cent, the retinol content is quite high, but it is combined with nourishing ingredients, such as passionfruit, apricot, kale, winter cherry extracts, skin-firming peptides and essential fatty acids. This means you can have all the benefits – even skin tone, bouncier skin, dramatically diminished wrinkles and fine lines – without the fear of irritation. The only thing that might cause irritation is the price. But it is definitely one worth paying.

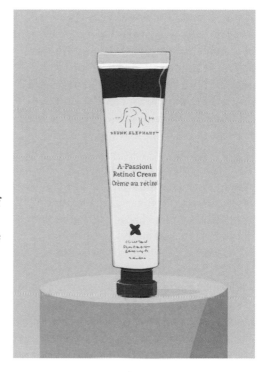

BEAUTY PIE™
Über Youth™ Re-Elastic Concentrate Serum

While Beauty Pie tout this as 'the closest thing we've found to a face lift in a bottle', it was not the possibility of getting a surprised face with eyebrows pulled up into the middle of my forehead that wooed me – I can achieve that by getting a fresh head of box braids. No, it was the divine scent. In my past life, I would never have gone for anything like this. Like many women who have been dealing with pigmentation issues for ever, you automatically make a beeline for the products that keep that in check and ignore the rest. This does not bode well – skin needs hydration, plumping, elasticity, refining … woman cannot live by bread alone, and all that. I have had to train my brain to experiment with skincare products and not just dark-spot destroyers and that's why I gave this a try. It claims to be firming and lifting but ignore that – I always find those terms utterly meaningless. It also says it reshapes your face. I don't know. My face shape looks just as round as it did when I started; so perhaps we ignore that, too. Here is the useful stuff you need to know: it has brilliant smoothing capabilities – this is the difference between youthful and decrepit skin. The infusion of the Double-Moisture Plus, essentially a super-hydrating complex that includes hyaluronic acid and other clever stuff, will make your skin look plumped and healthy. It's the kind of skin you see on people who live wonderful lives surrounded by sublime air quality. This serum also contains a red clover extract, which hydrates as well as smooths the skin, a liquorice extract, which is amazing for brightening, and a pine bark extract that boosts moisture in the skin. If you read the blurb on the packaging, it does say it is for Normal/Dehydrated to Dry Skin, but I reckon you can also use it on oilier skin types, because while it is rich – but non-sticky/greasy – it is not heavy, and it delivers deep-dive hydration, which also helps to balance oiliness. And then, of course, there's the fact that it smells SO nice.

CAUDALIE
Vinoperfect Radiance Serum

I've created (in my head) a beauty category called 'I'd drink it if I could'. I feel this way about Caudalie's Vinoperfect Radiance Serum. I use it post cleanser and liquid exfoliator, and for anyone dealing with dark spots and dull, greying skin that looks like it's been in an ash storm, it is an utter treat. On the back of my love for this serum, I have bought other products within this much-loved brand, but nothing else has quite hit the spot. It's like buying a very hyped album and discovering you only really like that one song (for me it was *Songs in A Minor* by Alicia Keys). The issue is that this serum has set the bar so high. When I stumbled upon it, years ago, I gave it a try, hoping something would come out of it. I am, like anyone contending with an uneven skin tone, forever seeking the Holy Grail of solutions. The results far exceeded my expectations. It smooths and brightens skin (the glow is off the Richter scale), reduces the appearance of dark spots (including acne scarring and pregnancy marks) and prevents them from reappearing. What's even more impressive is that it does all this in epic timing: my skin looks better within days of using this. The miracle ingredient is the patented Viniferine. This highly concentrated concoction is 62 times more effective than vitamin C at boosting radiance and evening out the complexion. The consistency is also a point scorer. The colour is reminiscent of the unctuous condensed milk many kids in Nigeria were obsessed with in the 1980s, but the texture is satin thin and absorbs beautifully into the skin. If I had any gripes about this product it would be that the price has slowly but surely increased over the years, and that the bottle finishes way too quickly. The latter, to be fair, isn't the brand's fault. It's down to my over zealous 'why use one drop when you can use ten?'. And perhaps, somewhere in my dreams, I am secretly drinking it.

MARIO BADESCU
Skin Care Facial Spray

In my opinion, most of the facial sprays and mists on the market are an overpriced swizz. However, if you are sold on one, I would advise that you avoid ones which cost a fortune and hone in on those that go beyond the 'refresh', such as Mario Badescu's facial spray range. The mist comes in four colours: orange, which tones and clears skin; purple, which includes vitamin C so is great for brightening; pink, the original cult favourite that works well on really dehydrated skin; and green, which is calming, antioxidant-rich, and acts like a wake-up call for lacklustre skin (and sometimes for me when I'm grumpy, tired and tempted to go back to bed). They are all non-greasy, balancing and suitable for sensitive skin. They are also great to use before or after applying your moisturiser to boost your skin's hydration levels, which is why they tend to be ubiquitous in make-up artists' kits. However, whilst one of the by-products of hydrated skin is that your make-up does sit and keep better, this won't work as a setting spray. Just keep that in mind and you won't be disappointed.

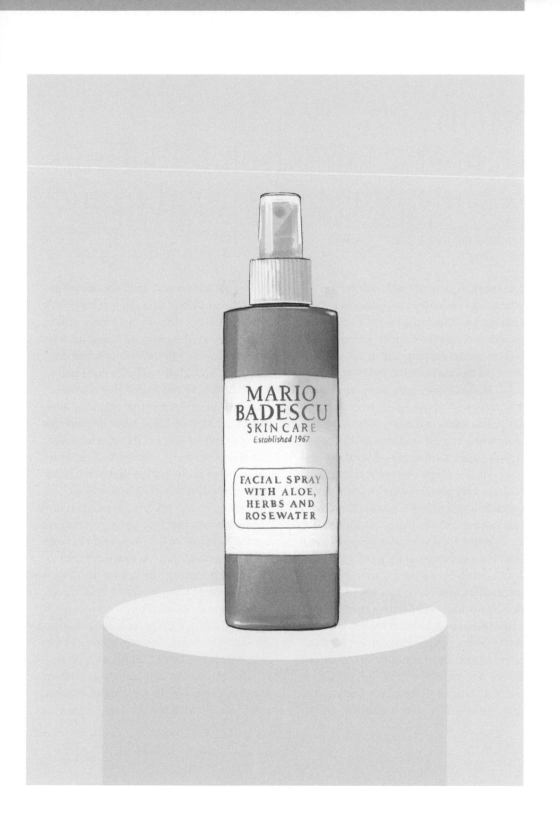

NIOD
Copper Amino Isolate Serum & Multi-Molecular Hyaluronic Complex

Laziness, like procrastination I've realised, is a bit like scrolling on Instagram at midnight. All enemies of progress. I had the Copper Amino Isolate Serum on my desk for a little bit (OK, it was months) before I used it. And you know why? Because the name was convoluted. Because the box was fiddly to open. Because I was too much in a hurry to bother. And then when I finally got around to opening it, I saw that it came in two bottles – one a serum, the other a mixer/activator-type thing – a bit like those careful-it-might-explode home hair-dying kits. Well, that just tipped me over the edge, and I left it to gather dust for a few more months. I will wait hours in a queue for a sample sale, I will spend ages scouting for a Pret in an unfamiliar area, because only they make croissants and cappuccinos exactly how I like them, and I have been known to sit for 13 hours getting the teeniest perfect braids done. But I couldn't be bothered to take a few seconds to mix the contents of two tiny bottles that had the potential to give me amazing skin, because it felt too

much like hard work. The turning point was when I visited a facialist at the Pfeffer Sal studios. My skin was in a state of flux. It was uneven, breaking out, and it looked as miserable as I felt. As she worked on my skin, the facialist asked me if I had heard of this serum by NIOD. Oh, yes, I replied, breezily, it is sitting on my desk, but I haven't used it yet. She revealed that the contents of that bottle were actually the answer to many, if not all, of my skin woes. It is a multi-tasker that penetrates deeply into the skin cells and targets numerous issues: textural damage, uneven pigmentation, enlarged pores, premature ageing, and loss of firmness and radiance. Copper peptides have antioxidant and anti-inflammatory properties, and they are found naturally in the skin, but as we age, they decrease. This serum counteracts this by encouraging skin to look and act younger (that is, the plump, bouncy, blemish-free skin we all had before we became acne-riddled teenagers). She then worked it on my skin as part of the treatment. I looked in the mirror afterwards, and my skin had been transformed. Gone was the congestion bubbling beneath my pores; the surface of my skin was smooth and even, and everything just glowed. Yes, of course, the actual facial boosted the results, but even using a few drops after your daily cleanser the results are tangible – you can expect to see better skin in five days. Layer it with NIOD's Multi-Molecular Hyaluronic Complex, and don't be surprised if people stop you in the street to ask for your skincare regime. The hyaluronic acid is hands down one of the very best on the market. Yes, they all technically do the same thing: they hold 1,000 times their weight in moisture and impart ridiculous levels of hydration to the skin. But they are not all equal. NIOD's is a much cleverer formulation that boosts the skin's moisture levels really quickly. The texture is much weightier and definitely has more depth than its cheaper counterparts, because the complex is an amalgamation of 15 different types of hyaluronic acid. So it may be more expensive than your standard product, but totally justified.

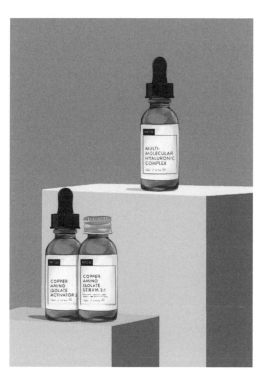

MASKS

THINGS TO NOTE...

Unless you have a Eurocentric nose,
good luck getting a sheet mask to
fit. That's fine, because most are
overrated and with the advancement
of technologies and textures, plenty of
alternative masks – for every possible
skin concern – are killing it instead.

EVE LOM
Rescue Mask

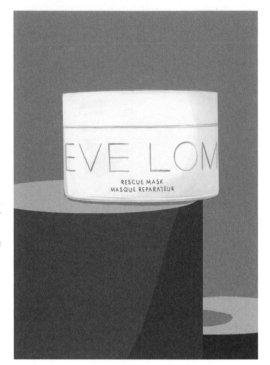

As a teenager, there were a couple of things that made me think life as an adult could not come soon enough. Like the fact my father would no longer be in the position to ban me from going raving with my friends because 'you can just put on the radio and dance in your room'. I also thought I would no longer have to deal with zits. I was right about the former, but oh, so wrong about the latter. This is where the Rescue Mask comes in. It is a putty white mix of camphor, honey, kaolin clay and almonds – these are the exfoliating particles you'll notice peppered through the mask (it looks like a really thick Oreo milkshake). At a time when sheet masks are all the rage, a mask you slather on your face, somewhat chaotically, probably feels quite retro. I don't mind that at all. I don't really rate those Phantom of the Opera-style sheet masks, give me a good old-school mask any day. This paste goes on quite thickly; so, you can expect it to last a while. You do feel a cooling, tingling sensation when it goes on and as it begins to dry, you start to see your pores through it. At that point it is decongesting (that's the camphor at work) and absorbing any excess oil (kaolin clay) without stripping it (thank you, honey). I tend to leave it on for about 15 minutes and then rinse off. One thing to note about the rinsing aspect – it can get really messy, and it's not a one-rinse job. Use a muslin cloth, otherwise you'll find bits of it in and around your nose and hairline. These are the perils of clay masks. But consider the pros: your skin is immediately clearer and brighter, the raging breakouts bubbling under your skin calm right down, and your pores look so clean you could eat off them.

HERBIVORE
Blue Tansy Resurfacing Clarity Mask

The first thing that attracted me to this mask is the fact that it is blue. Alas, it doesn't look blue on your skin. Instead it dries to a clear, 'glass skin' finish, so there go your hopes of starring in the Avatar sequel. The second thing that drew me to it was its minimalist jar: I like nice fonts and clean, white spaces, and I have been known to forgo a product on the basis of packaging that induces a migraine. In this case, thankfully, substance over style rules the roost – this mask really does perform, and I have been harping on about it to anyone who cares to listen. Unfortunately, however, no one could actually get hold of it, because it turns out that it didn't meet EU regulations. Thankfully, the US-based brand managed to get its act together so that we could get this little miracle worker on this side of the Atlantic. Expect clearer, smoother and brighter skin, which, amazingly, is immediately visible (can you tell I have no patience for slow burners?).

The star ingredient, blue tansy oil, which is what gives this product its hue, is great for soothing dry skin. But this is not one of my problems; quite the opposite, in fact: my skin could win awards for its oil-producing capabilities. What I do suffer from, however, is dehydrated skin, and this does help my skin look more hydrated, less like a road map. Other key ingredients are white willow bark – naturally high in salicin which clarifies acne-prone skin – and fruit enzymes, such as pineapple and papaya, which exfoliate the skin and resurface the complexion. The watery gel-like texture is a little messy to apply but that aside, it is everything you could want from a mask. And for all the nice fonts and shades of blue, that's really what counts.

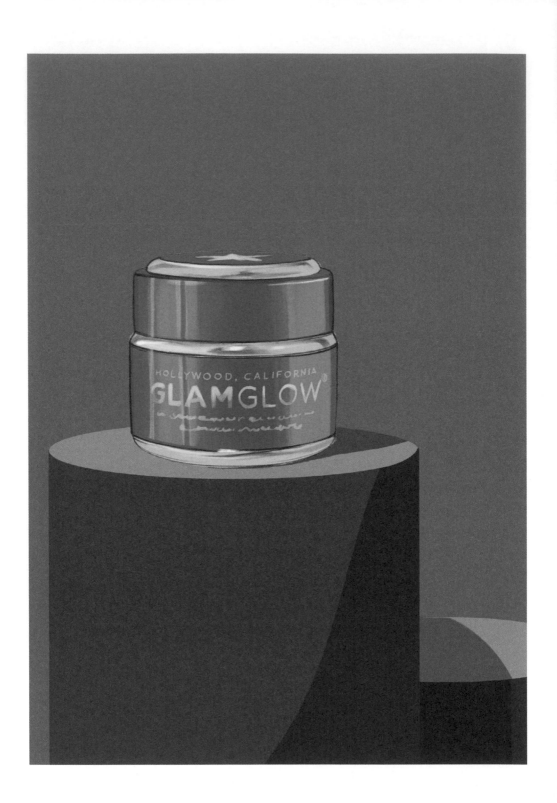

GLAMGLOW
Flashmud™ Brightening
Treatment

Before I met my husband, I found going on dates utterly torturous. I have a friend who also consistently experienced rubbish dates, but whereas I left most praying they lost my number, every so often she'd give one of her terrible dates a second chance. One turned out to be a good move; ten years later they are still together, madly in love and expecting what seems like their 75th child. I was never that kind of girl, and I long applied a similar ethos to my beauty products. The first time I used this mask, I didn't like it at all. I found the box fiddly to open and was irritated that it was way too big for the small pot it housed – too much packaging is a bugbear of mine, and many beauty brands are still so out of step on this. The fact is, we had kicked off on the wrong foot, and so I smeared it on with disdain, left it for 5 minutes, then rinsed it off. I didn't feel interested enough to pay attention to what effect, if any, it might have had. However, when I went back to it some weeks later, I kind of fell in love. I noticed things I hadn't noticed before. For a start, it smells lovely; a very subtle, fresh fruitiness. The ingredients in this include willow bark, white jasmine flower and white birch leaf, all of which make up a multi-brightening complex that

works to reduce dark spots, dullness and an uneven skin tone; if these are your skin issues, this pot of magic is an essential. Initially the texture looks thick and creamy, but on closer inspection it is more like a speckled, whipped mousse. Now, I'll take an acid liquid exfoliator over a physical one any day; however, the grains here are ground so finely they won't damage the skin. The key is to massage gently, not scrub; remember, your face is not a cooking pot. The directions state you leave it on for a minimum of 20 minutes and for good reason – less time than this, and you'll get half-hearted results. They also say that the mask will begin to look translucent on the skin. Er, it didn't. I found that it stayed pretty much opaque. No matter, because once I rinsed off with warm water my skin looked incredible – brighter, clearer and luminous. Dark spots were much less visible, and my skin was smoother and more even. Your serums will also be better absorbed, your make-up will sit better, and you'll understand why everyone raves about this cult classic (it started life as a red-carpet favourite). And to think I had dismissed it! The moral of this story? Some bad first dates deserve a second chance.

PETER THOMAS ROTH
Cucumber Gel Mask

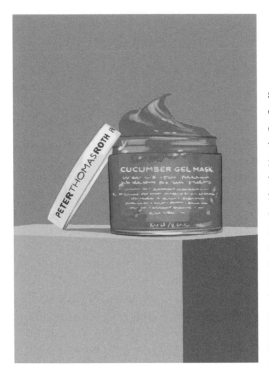

The cartoonishly green hue of this mask reminds me of the jellies you used to get at children's birthday parties. Most had artificial colours and even fewer natural ingredients, which is probably why we were all bouncing off the walls. The ingredients in this gel – cucumber, papaya, chamomile, pineapple, orange, lemon – have a much more positive impact. Now, let's be clear, if you are simply looking for a mask to deal with hyperpigmentation or clearing congestion then this is not it. It is ideal for dry and dehydrated skin types and skin that is very sensitive. But even if you don't fit into those skin types, please don't dismiss this. There is a good reason one of these is sold globally every minute. This mask is all about hydration, of which every type of skin needs a good dose to look and function at its optimal level. I love the light cucumber-scented gel, which goes on clear and instantly feels incredibly cooling. This doesn't sound like much but try using it on holiday after a day at the beach; your skin will drink it up. It is the perfect hot-weather/sunburnt-skin companion – yes, people, black does crack, and it definitely burns. After about 10–15 minutes, rinse it off and you will notice your skin looks more hydrated and less sore. While hydration is the gel's primary function, it also tightens pores, works as an antioxidant to protect against free radicals and improves luminosity. If you are the kind of person happy to add another step to your already trillion-step regime you can use this daily (it is tremendous as an overnight mask). Otherwise 2–3 times a week should suffice. As I said, this is not a shouty hardcore mask that claims to destroy the forces of evil advancing on your skin, but the results will have you bouncing off walls; in a good way.

CHARLOTTE TILBURY
Goddess Skin Clay Mask

This is a great mask. Actually, let me caveat that. The greatness of a mask is really down to what it promises and what your expectations are. If you have had a stress-induced breakout on the eve of a big, important, 'everyone will be there' event, this mask will not help you. If you are in the market for softer, smoother skin and pores that don't gape like the back of a badly fitting pair of jeans, then carry on reading. I will admit that historically I have been a little sceptical about make-up brands that delve into skincare, but this supercharged mask is noteworthy. It uses kaolin clay to draw out impurities and a peptide complex to hydrate and plump up the skin. It is perfect if your skin looks fatigued and congested and the texture a little, dare I say it, rough. I like the fact that it is in a tube and not a tub: the potential for bacterial transference is lessened. The mask is a pale peach hue that reminds me of a colour from a posh paint brand, and it smells divine – like a retro powder compact. The texture of this mask will also tick boxes: it is creamy and malleable, so never goes concrete hard. You are supposed to follow the Charlotte Tilbury Wonder Workout Massage Technique online and leave it on for 10 minutes. Do I think this is necessary? Not really, but, hey, if you have the time, knock yourself out. After rinsing, you will notice brighter, cleaner, softer skin with less visible pores, as opposed to the lacklustre mess you were dealing with pre-mask. For oilier skin types, everything immediately looks more balanced and your make-up will go on like a dream. Just don't get it in your eyes, because it stings. A lot.

DR SEBAGH
Deep Exfoliating Mask

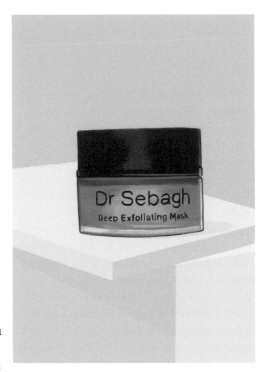

I used trillions of masks when I was a teenager, and they were all rubbish. I had to resist the urge to weep with disappointment every time I rinsed one off and saw my skin looked exactly as it had 20 minutes prior. If only I'd had this magical orange beauty all those years ago. If you are waging war with dull, discoloured, blemish-prone skin, this is a gift. The purpose of the potent formula (which includes azelaic, glycolic and lactic acids) is to exfoliate deep into the pores and resurface the skin. It does that and more: it is a facial in a jar. The whipped orange concoction does smell a bit science lab – you almost expect a smoky sulphuric cloud to appear and hover over it. It's a no-nonsense, playtime-is-over, 'we mean business' kind of mask. Admittedly, years ago, I found this rather intimidating, but my desperation for better skin was stronger than the fear that my face might fall off. Once you apply the orange paste, which comes with a little applicator, you feel what I can only describe as a kind of sizzling. I imagine it's a bit like having tiny piranhas nibbling away at your dead skin. OK, it's not that horrendous, but it is pretty tingly, hence the advice on the label for first-timers to take it off after 3–5 minutes. Use it regularly, and you'll probably be able to extend this. Still, be it 5 or 15 minutes, the results are phenomenal and instantaneous. Now, let's be clear: if you're seeking a soothing, pampering kind of situation, you're on the wrong bus. If your skin type is sensitive, there is a sensitive version available. But if you need a problem-skin solution or a radiance-boosting pre-party treatment, this does not fall short. And, yes, it is not dirt cheap; I was a badly paid assistant when I first became obsessed and it was terrible for my bank balance. But, incredible for my skin.

ORIGINS
Clear Improvement™
Active Charcoal Mask

Sometimes I find the obsession with newness in the beauty industry a little tiresome. Not everything new is great, not everything aesthetically elaborate is worth the box it comes in and not everything old should be discarded. This mask has been around for a while; it is clay based, does not really fit into the Instagrammable-product category and dries so tight your face may as well be in a straitjacket. Pretty old school. But who cares? The formulation is fabulous. The charcoal, white clay and lecithin in the mask act like a magnet that sucks out all the pollution, debris, bacteria and general dirt congregating in your pores. Nice. Perhaps think of it as a vacuum for your face. The smell, mild and charcoal-like (obviously), is forgettable, in the best possible way. 15 minutes in, the creamy texture dries. Your face then feels taut but, surprisingly, doesn't crack; you just look ridiculous, and find it challenging to speak. After rinsing off, you will notice three things: your skin looks really, really clean and feels incredibly smooth, and you will look lit from within. Which I think is rather unusual, and special, for an old-school clay mask.

REN
Clean Skincare Glycol Lactic Radiance Renewal Mask

This mask sloughs off dead skin cells, unplugs congested pores and combats blemishes. Essentially, it is a triumph, and if you have problematic skin, it should be a key part of your beauty stash. So, what else do you need to know? Well, it is orange; a sedate Berocca-tablet orange as opposed to the acidic sort that glows in the dark. It is also unusually sticky. This might not go down well with everyone. I have heard some people say the mask is so sticky that their hands stick to their faces. That is a ridiculous exaggeration – the texture is closer to an adhesive-like stickiness; it's not superglue. Anyway, you can't please everyone. The scent, however, a pleasant orange, is unlikely to be as divisive. Still, don't let the prettiness of the hue and the lovely smell fool you: this is still quite a hardcore mask (not appropriate for sensitive skins), and once it goes on, it tingles. This is generally the case with anything that has acids such as glycolic and lactic in the mix. What you feel on your skin is the acids breaking down the dead layers of your skin. While this doesn't sound particularly inviting, personally I love acids. They will refine, resurface and revamp, and all darker skin tones should incorporate them into their regime. Ideally, use this at night and follow it with an overnight liquid exfoliator and some hyaluronic acid for incredible results.

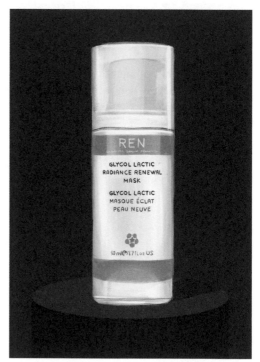

SISLEY
Black Rose Cream Mask

It costs a fortune, and it is 60ml. Even if you are appalling at maths, you only have to look at it to know this is an eye-watering investment. I remember thinking this was a sample size but, no, it's the real deal. As beauty editors we can be quite spoilt for choice, and so we have to be careful not to fall into a bubble, where our sense of prices becomes totally warped. It is not cheap by any standards. But, oh, it is amazing. Years ago, I resisted this mask for two reasons. First, the price. I don't believe you should start using a product you can't realistically afford to keep up with. It's like buying a fancy car on credit then never having enough money to fill up the tank. Second, everyone who swore by it was white, so I just didn't believe it would have any real impact on my skin. I am now, however, a fully paid-up member of the Black Rose Club. You will notice that the front of the packaging says 'Instant Youth'. This type of hyperbolic claim would normally irk me – because, let's face it, no such thing exists – but I actually get what they mean. This Black Rose smooths and plumps, and makes you look less defeated by life.

In addition to the vitamin B_5, shea butter and padina pavonica – all 'anti-agers' – it does make you look more youthful. Unsurprisingly, everything about this product is luxe. The scent, a rich rose, is the authentic, exquisite, expensive stuff – not the weird chemical compound you get in low-rent candles. The texture is more akin to applying an expensive night cream than a traditional mask. It initially looks white, but within minutes it is completely translucent, and your face appears drenched in a clear liquid highlighter. After rinsing off, your skin is most definitely, visibly plumper and smoother. The product blurb does say that it also brightens, and while I agree that you will look more luminous, I wouldn't specifically recommend it for pigmentation issues. You need something more targeted for that. Yet, for skin that is lethargic, mature, dehydrated or just needs an injection of life, this is glorious. And highly addictive. And expensive. But so good. It's a slippery slope. Feel free to join me.

ALPHA-H
Liquid Gold™ Ultimate Perfecting Mask

I have a soft spot for this mask.
I discovered it years ago when I was going through a really challenging time with my skin. As with so many of the brands I have discovered and fallen in love with, it all began with a facial. I had heard the Alpha-H facial was great for congestion, hyperpigmentation and scarring. Back then most facials were mainly about 'rejuvenating' and 'refreshing' – words that were meaningless in terms of their effects. Also, they were very much targeting white skin and struggled to make any difference to mine. It was a breath of fresh air to discover a facial that could potentially work on women of colour. As I made the long journey to the clinic, I hoped no one would see me – my skin was in such a state. Post treatment, I looked in the mirror and welled up at how much clearer, brighter and decongested it looked, as if a whole layer of dead, speckled skin had been taken off, and my breakouts were diminished. This mask, used within my facial, was pivotal to my radical transformation. You could call it an advanced peel, but that might sound a bit scary – a peel conjures images of a face that looks like a raw chicken and

needs emergency treatment. Instead, think of it as a supercharged exfoliating treatment that clears congestion, lifts dead skin cells, regulates sebum production, evens out skin tone, increases collagen production and boosts hydration levels. Yep, it is a mask that gives you facial-like results without having to leave the comfort of your own bathroom. The silky white consistency doesn't dry like concrete, but neither does it remain creamy. It lies somewhere in between. It is acid based – glycolic, lactic and ferulic acids – and so, yes, it does sting a little but not so much you run around screaming because your face is on fire. Besides, you only need to keep it on for 10 minutes. Some acid-based masks can make the skin feel a little taut, but what's great about this one is that it draws moisture to the surface of the skin, so it feels really hydrated. The formulation has changed since the original, and I'll admit when I noticed this, my heart sank. Reformulations have a habit of being a poor imitation of the original. But I was pleasantly surprised. It is every bit as brilliant as it was when we first met.

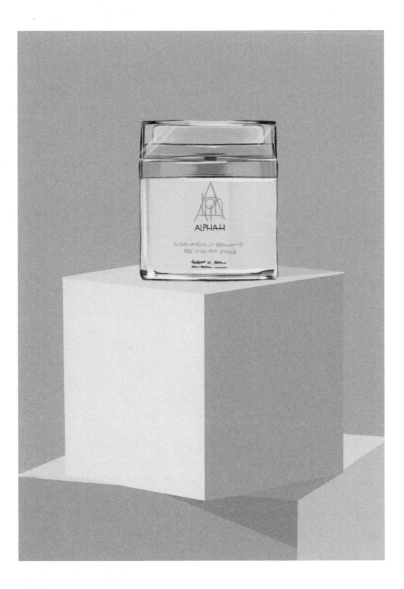

S U N C A R E

THINGS TO NOTE...

Hurrah! I have unearthed sunscreens
free of the white cast, many of
which will treat your pigmentation
while preventing any more from
forming. You can also wear them
under make-up without the fear that
your pores will be clogged up with
gunk. No more excuses: get a sunscreen
and use it regularly, because dark skins
do burn and not just on the beach.

COOLA
Classic Sport Face
SPF 50 White Tea

I have harped on about this sunscreen so much, I'm sure people think I secretly work for Coola. I just love it; it ticks so many boxes. Most obviously, it doesn't leave that 'Oh, my God, it's a ghost' look. The 'Face Sport' element in the product name is probably a bit confusing. It is, according to the website blurb, for people who want to 'live their best life' (honestly, who writes this stuff?) and is geared towards those who live a very active lifestyle by being sweat and water resistant for up to 80 minutes. This gives me visions of women with thighs to rival Serena Williams's, who worship at the altar of their local gym and do their food shop while wearing leggings and a matching crop top. That woman is not me. I don't own any Spandex. Spin classes are my idea of modern-day torture, and my Gazelles have never seen the inside of a gym. But never mind that I'm not their target audience, it works. I love the scent – white tea – and the light, creamy texture. It gives a luminous finish that is rare for an SPF 50 formulation, which, traditionally, slathers on like a white sludge. Another thing that sets it apart from many of its counterparts is that it is more than just sun protection: the evening primrose oil, linseed oil and safflower oleosomes are brilliant antioxidants and hydrators.

A few points to note. Some may find the finish a bit oily. I personally think it's more a dewiness, but if you prefer a matte look, this might not be the best option. Another criticism is that it is a bit slippery under make-up. Fair point. I suggest using a pea-size amount and waiting at least 5 minutes before applying foundation. As with all sunscreens, there is one glaring issue. After 2–3 hours, whatever sunscreen you applied before leaving home, you know, the one that promised to protect you against wrinkles, sun damage, dark spots and cancer, will disappear. This is why all sunscreen brands tell you to reapply every couple of hours. When you already have a full face of make-up on, this is a problem. Thankfully, Coola also produces a **Makeup Setting Spray** that you can spritz throughout the day, which comes with an inbuilt SPF 30. Problem sorted.

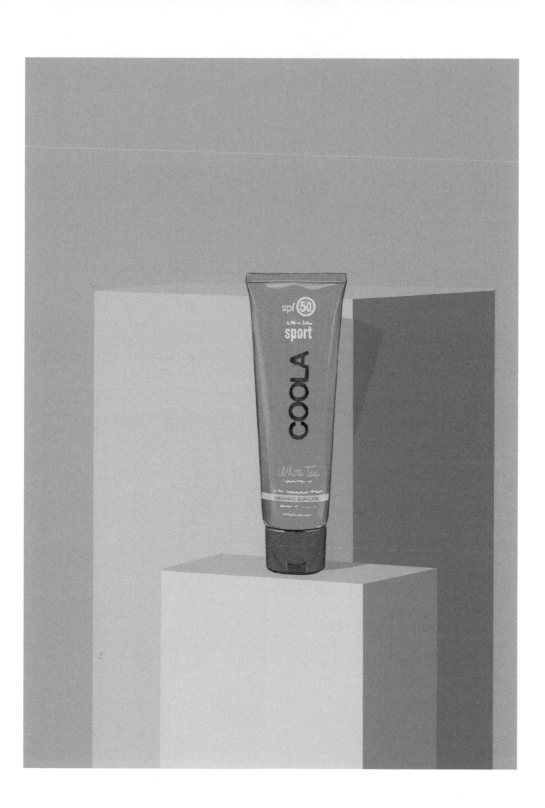

BY TERRY
UV Base Sunscreen Cream Broad Spectrum SPF 50

In the past I've questioned make-up brands that think they can also authentically 'own' skincare. Can you really do it all? Can you? Yes, I know we are in the age of the hyphenate and everything, and I'm not trying to kill anyone's dream here, but there is wisdom in being true to what you do best, 'staying in your lane' as it were. But not always. By Terry (the brand launched by Terry de Gunzburg, the genius behind Yves Saint Laurent's cult classic, Touche Éclat) is one of the few make-up brands where the quality and tech of the skincare is on a par with many of the bigger players on the market. This sunscreen is excellent, a glossy hybrid between a cream and a serum that doesn't leave a white trace. It is neither matte nor oily – somewhere in between – and so works well as a skin-smoothing make-up primer. What Terry de Gunzburg famously does is create products that are steeped in complex, technologically advanced formulations, and she has nailed it here. It is highly

unusual to find an SPF 50 that has really great skincare properties – hydrating, anti-pollution, vitamin E – while remaining incredibly lightweight (many traditional SPF 50s will give you a helping of blackheads). I love the fact that it has a delightful fragrance, but as it's not cheap, it is simply good manners to smell nice.

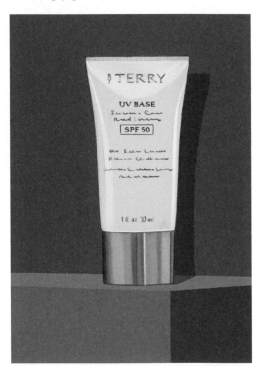

SISLEY
Super Soin Solaire Youth Protector Face SPF 50+

Unless you are drunk or feeling particularly generous because you have suddenly come into money, this is the sunscreen you should probably never share. I know, it's not particularly magnanimous, but one look at the price and you'll see why not everything in life falls under the 'sharing-is-caring' mantra. This is the crème de la crème of sunscreens and like all Sisley products, it is not a snip. So why pay the price? Well, it is like couture, the quality is sublime. It does a myriad of things: protects the skin from oxidative stress (this is the principal cause of photo ageing, which includes wrinkles, hyperpigmentation and dehydration), reduces fine lines and minimises the look of dark spots. It works on the skin at a cellular level, which, in layman's terms, means it stops your skin from building up so many dead layers that people begin to mistake you for a rhino. The edelweiss and camellia-oil extract allow your skin to maintain its optimum hydration levels, and because it also includes shea butter and mango extract, your skin is smoother and more supple. All this comes without the grey finish and pore-clogging powers sunscreens normally wield. The cream-like formulation might be slightly misleading; it does look quite dense, but it rubs into the skin without leaving that unsightly tinge. The sage and marjoram scent is faint and disappears in seconds. And so will the entire contents of this tube if you don't use restraint. I apply that same philosophy to the 'body' equivalent – **Super Soin Solaire Youth Protector Milky Body Mist SPF 30** – which I have used for years, and when I say years, I mean I wheel out the same bottle every summer holiday. Somewhere in my heart I am guessing it has long expired, but you know what, I haven't burnt, it hasn't curdled, it still smells fine (lavender and geranium – bliss), and I haven't broken out in hives. Yes, it is teeny and pricey, but apply it like a miser, never share it, it'll last a lifetime.

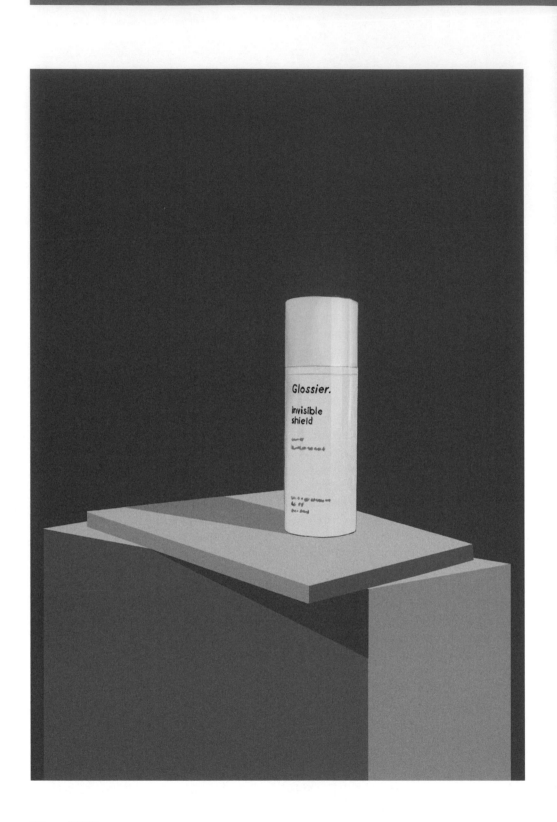

GLOSSIER
Invisible Shield Daily Sunscreen SPF 35

I'd like to think that as a long-in-the-tooth beauty editor, I'm so incredibly grounded (read: jaded) that I am immune to the hype of a new brand or launch. But, of course, that's utter rubbish. Case in point: Glossier. A few years ago, I visited the Glossier offices and store in New York and had a field day trying and buying products, picking up all the branded postcards, taking lots of footage for social media and asking the staff where I could buy the pale pink jumpsuits they all had on – it was the coolest 'uniform' I had seen for a while. I was like a kid in a candy shop. And then when the brand finally hit the UK, like everyone else, I went into hyperventilating mode. I got everything and anything. I even got the sweatshirt. The point is I love Glossier. But do I use all the range? Embarrassingly, no. Not very much of it. I love the idea of Glossier. I love that it is lovely to look at. I love the ethos. I love the authentic sense of community they have created, and I love the clever forward-thinking way they operate – no one else was asking their followers what

sort of cleanser they should launch or what they should name it. But I think Glossier is essentially for those who like a simplistic, barely there aesthetic, and that isn't really me.

There is one product in the Glossier line-up that I use more than anything else: the sunscreen (yes, I know sunscreen is not 'sexy', but then neither is skin cancer). It is superb, and, notably, invisible, as the name states. The texture is a water-gel formula that reminds me a little of their **Milky Jelly Cleanser**, except it smells of sweet oranges and blends easily into skin. Yes, this includes black skin. Not only does it protect the skin from the sun's rays, the ingredients list – vitamin E, broccoli and aloe leaf – reads like an ode to antioxidants. It is not chalky, sticky, greasy or sunscreen-y; the founder, ex-*Vogue* journalist Emily Weiss, touts it as the sunscreen for people who don't like to wear sunscreen. Which, alas, includes 99 per cent of the black women I know. So here you go. It is everything you didn't think a sunscreen could be.

NYDG
Chem-Free Active Defense SPF 30

This has been created by a group of well-regarded New York dermatologists (hence the name, New York Dermatology Group). I trust dermatologists and I can tell you that the formulation behind this sunscreen is bona-fide. Now, I will admit, I was a little perplexed when I initially squeezed some of the product out of the tube; it was like watching a snail move in slow motion. Then there's the colour and stiff texture – bicarbonate-of-soda white and cement thick. I couldn't understand how something supposedly 'lightweight' and 'great for sensitive skin' had a density that could surface roads. But looks are deceiving. No, it doesn't behave like a gel consistency, which tends to disappear immediately, but once you begin to rub it into the skin (you don't need much) you realise it is permeable and does not leave you ashy. One of the ingredients is zinc oxide, and the majority of sunscreens I have tried that include this leave a chalky residue. The fact that this sunscreen does not is testament to the superiority of the formula. Another plus point is that it contains squalane and argan oils, so acts like an antioxidant and hydrating moisturiser. While oilier skins may baulk at the idea of anything with oil, this leaves skin with a non-sticky finish. It is also unscented (sensitive skins will love it) and can be used on the body. The physicians behind it are athletic types who love to surf, hence, for 80 minutes, it is also water and sweat resistant. Target audience? People with really active lifestyles. And, no, the time you spend perfecting your posts and engaging with your followers on social media doesn't count.

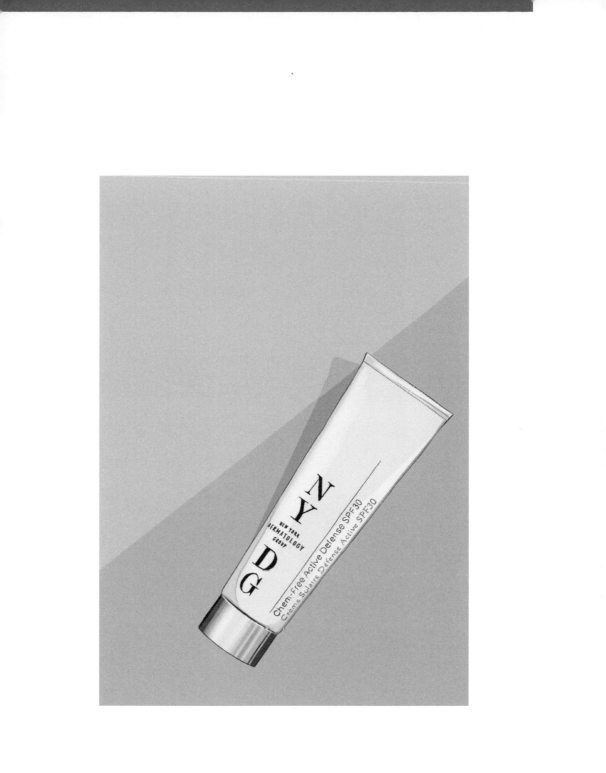

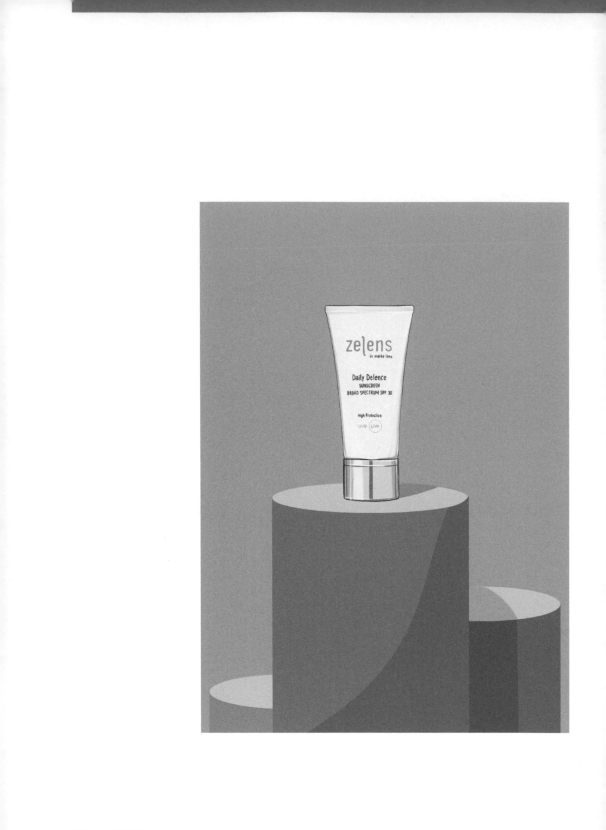

ZELENS
Daily Defence Sunscreen Broad Spectrum SPF 30

Years ago, I was researching a feature where I was trying to find the SPFs that wouldn't cause flashback in photography. (The 'flashback' kind of SPF is where the camera makes you look as if you've been bathed in calamine lotion. This happens to both dark and Caucasian skin tones – who says the beauty industry isn't inclusive?) Finding 'anti-flashback' sunscreens meant a long and hard search, testing what felt like a million of them. Generally speaking, I discovered that those which fell under the 'chemical sunscreens' banner (as opposed to 'physical' sunscreens, which contain titanium dioxide and sit on top of the skin) are less likely to leave a white cast. At the time, Zelens Daily Defence was the best I found, and it still is one of the very best available. It was one of the few that didn't have that polarising sunscreen scent or a vicious smell, like something concocted in the dark lab of an evil dictator. Instead it is probably the nicest-smelling sunscreen I've come across. Alas, many of these high-performing sunscreens that work well on darker skin tones tend to be on the higher end of the price scale. While the high street is flooded with a plethora of sunscreen brands at pocket-friendly prices, most I've tried would only come in handy if I were

auditioning for the lead role in *Casper the Friendly Ghost*. I do think this sunscreen is worth its high price, however. I'll try not to bore you with the science, but what we have here is a super-astute and innovative micro-encapsulation technology giving you an intense level of sun protection. With this, your skin is able to deflect the sun's rays, while the antioxidants help repair existing damage. It includes hyaluronic acid, which plumps up the skin, vitamin C to brighten hyperpigmentation and it stimulates the production of collagen – the stuff that stops your skin looking like a flat tyre. There is a lot of impressive stuff going on in this tube. It won't interfere with your make-up and can be used on any skin – including sensitive-skin types, who normally find sunscreens aggravating. At first I was a little concerned about the consistency (it is quite thick), but I found it eased into the skin like a silky day cream, and I promise it does not give you the dreaded 'I've just been dusted with self-raising flour' finish. So, feel free to tap into your narcissistic side and take all the selfies you want with this one. No filter required.

DR. BARBARA STURM
Sun Drops SPF 50

Years before these drops came on to the market, Dr Sturm, recognising that darker skin tones have unique challenges, launched a skincare line specifically for us. One of our skincare 'challenges' is our relatively limited choice of sunscreen, so I was surprised that this product didn't specifically mention its suitability for people of colour. Perhaps it was an oversight. I have to remind myself not to see a race issue where there is none. So, no, it doesn't say it specifically, but it is for us. The concept is rather innovative; you put a few drops in anything, and you have your sun protection. Actually, scrap that, you can't mix it in anything: I wouldn't recommend you put it in a juice and drink it, unless your life goal is getting your stomach pumped. When I say you can mix it in anything, I mean anything topical: creams, serums, moisturisers, even foundations and, *voilà*, you have your sun protection. Or as the founder says: 'It's your liquid sun umbrella'.

It has an unusual slip and the density of an upmarket custard, so you don't expect it to blend well, but it does so beautifully and seamlessly. There are also really great skin benefits – vitamin E and cassia extract promote skin-cell regeneration and work really well as intense hydrators. But I wouldn't recommend using it on its own. It is incredibly concentrated, and without another base to blend with, it can feel a bit like you've rubbed a sticky bun all over your face. But use it properly and it's a dream.

BEAUTY PIE™
Ultralight UVA/UVB SPF 25

There is quite a lot of Beauty Pie in this book. I love the brand. So many clever products with brilliant formulations and inclusive prices. This is yet another. First, I am in love with the aesthetic. The shape, the beautifully clean, minimalist design, the font ... Yes, I am a nerd who likes a bit of eye candy on her beauty shelf. Good packaging is good for the soul. In the grand scheme of things, however, those elements are not the most important – the quality of the sunscreen is. And it is outstanding. The silky, lightweight texture really does feel as if you are wearing nothing on your skin, which, I'm sure, is music to the ears of everyone with recurring pore-clogger nightmares. Then I love the fact that it has ingredients such as hyaluronic acid (renowned, of course, for its moisture-boosting superpowers) and liquorice extract. Now as much as I gag at the thought of liquorice-flavoured anything (I still can't believe there are people who voluntarily eat Liquorice Allsorts), there is no denying the incredible skincare benefits

for darker skin tones. Back in the day, I used a (sadly, long discontinued) mask that was infused with liquorice extracts, and it was the most amazing brightener. Another point scorer here is that this sunscreen is made in Japan. This fills me with confidence for two reasons: the technology behind Japanese beauty products is ahead of the curve, and the Japanese are obsessed with protecting their skin from the sun. It's a first-rate product that works for all skin types, plus the velvety finish means it is also brilliant as a pre-foundation primer. It has a very faint scent – quite floral and, thankfully, not liquorice. I have stints of travelling a lot for work, so I always value a light and dinky multi-tasker such as this. If you are the kind of person who likes to carry everything in her oversized, backache-inducing handbag for those 'what if' situations (you know, the ones that never, ever happen) the last thing you need is a sunscreen the size of a chihuahua.

BODY
DYE
CARE

THINGS TO NOTE...

Don't believe anyone who tells you great bodycare revolves around tech-driven products that promise to 'lift' or rid you of cellulite. It's a fallacy, they don't work, so please don't waste your money. The key to keeping your skin in tip-top condition is less convoluted. Simply approach it exactly as you would the skin on your face. Exfoliate (your moisturiser will work so much better), hydrate (the drier it is, the older it looks), protect (sunscreen: enough said) and every so often, treat it to an illuminator, the quickest way to revive lacklustre skin.

THE BODY SHOP®
Body Butters

This might sound odd, but I once had a friend with the shiniest of shins. If this *doesn't* sound odd to you, it's because you know that many people of colour are obsessed with keeping ashy skin at bay. At school, if your shins were dry, the ridicule you faced was acute, so needless to say, glistening shins were highly coveted. My shiny-shinned friend then revealed the secret to hers: Body Shop's Body Butters. I've been besotted with the range ever since. It is one of the absolute best on the market, which is an achievement, considering it is also one of the least expensive. Unlike traditionally dense butters, this doesn't require elbow grease to apply, it won't leave you slithery or attracting debris, and you won't find yourself perspiring like a heavyweight boxer mid-fight. It is also a world away from the modern incarnations of 'butters', which are in reality lightweight lotions that leave an unsatisfying matte finish. Rather, this thick, semi-solid marvel has a rich, creamy texture, absorbs easily, and leaves your skin feeling beautifully moisturised all day with just the right level of shine. It comes in a myriad of scents, even the Strawberry and Mango – notes I would normally find nauseating – are glorious. If your skin is incredibly dry, Hemp, beloved by numerous eczema sufferers, is excellent. If you prefer something with an understated scent, Shea Butter (using community traded shea butter from Ghana) is ideal. Whatever you choose, you can be sure of one thing: the joys of shiny shins.

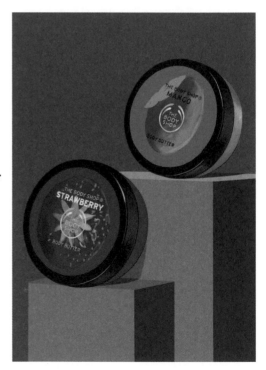

KIEHL'S
Crème de Corps

Over the years, I have tried a myriad of mainstream body lotions promising me everything but my hand in marriage. Cheap, expensive, mid price – you name it, they rarely come up to scratch. I realised, and sadly accepted, that the reason they didn't work was because the majority are created with Caucasian skins in mind, which generally respond better to much lighter lotions. I can't imagine recommending pure unrefined shea butter to any of my Caucasian friends, but for many of us, using unctuous body moisturisers daily that penetrate into skin and leave that head-to-toe coveted shine is a must. It's what we do to stop our bodies looking ashy. So when it comes to taste in lotions we are on opposite ends of the spectrum. Unless, of course, we are talking about Crème de Corps. I call it the UN of body moisturisers. It's not there to take sides and more or less everybody loves it. The buttery texture oozes like a lotion but has the fortitude of a cream. It is a neutral-scented blend of shea butter, avocado oil and squalane which keeps your skin soft, smooth, moisturised and ash-free all day. A mainstream modern-luxe body lotion that actually works on darker skin tones – something which shouldn't be ground breaking, but it is.

AMANDA HARRINGTON
Illuminating Bronzing Mousse

I have been open about the invites I've received over the years to 'come in for a fake tan' by brands who had neither bothered to check what colour I am, nor if they had products that suited my skin tone. To be fair, self-tanning wasn't a category I had been interested in exploring – until this came along. Brand founder Amanda Harrington is the tanning expert Oscar winners, music stars, high net worth individuals and fashion insiders have on their speed dial when they need a boost of colour. Because what Amanda does however is not what your run-of-the-mill spray tanners do. She brushes, blends and contours the skin with a concoction that leaves a magnificent but natural-looking, glow. She does exactly the same for darker skin tones because she understands that the desire for 'the glow' transcends race; only sea creatures aspire to grey skin.

Thankfully, you don't need to have her on speed dial yourself, because she has bottled her genius formulation in this frothy bronzy-gold mousse which you can apply at home. Once you've thoroughly exfoliated your body (and are hair free, sorry!) it is straightforward to apply. Use the kabuki-style brush sold alongside it to buff in the formula (which has smoothing and hydrating ingredients like hyaluronic acid, Q10 and collagen). Your coverage will be really even and it will last longer. Once you're done, you'll notice your glorious-looking body no longer resembles your face's poor relative. It's addictive and I'm now obsessed.

JO MALONE
Velvet Rose & Oud
Dry Body Oil

The lazy side of me loves moisturising with body oils, as they don't require the same effort necessary to work a cream into the skin. They also have the unrivalled ability to impart gloss and shine in a way that lotions could only dream of. Unfortunately, most have the same downside which is that once on, you have to wait a lifetime before you can get dressed. If you are already running late for an event and your dress is made of silk, this is a nuisance. Therefore, if you are set on oil, make it a dry oil. These are the clever, semi-skimmed sisters of your full-fat oils. They are not heavy – they have less slip than other oils – so they absorb easily into the skin without the dreaded greasy residue, making them perfect hot-weather fare. Jo Malone's version is my absolute favourite. Its practical, chic spray (numerous brands haven't quite read the memo that oils in a bottle with a gaping mouth is a stupid idea) allows you to control the output. Not high-shine, it is incredibly hydrating and the divine rose and oud scent means it can double up as perfume. An all-round win-win situation.

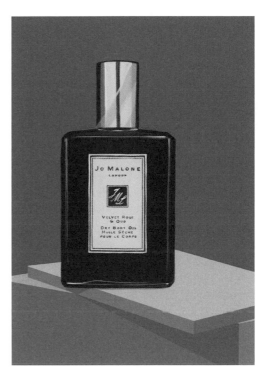

FENTY BEAUTY
Body Lava

Years ago, if you had told me I'd be the kind of human being who bothers with a body-highlighting product I would have laughed in your face. I like to think I'm too high-minded for that sort of stuff, but I now work in beauty, so really, who am I kidding? Besides, this product is sublime. The first time I used it, I thought about how much we neglect our bodies. We do everything to make sure our faces are always on point and then from the neck down, it's a 'poor cousin' syndrome. Once I clocked how much better my skin looked and felt – bronzy and incredibly soft, I was sold on the concept. This gel (in the shade Brown Sugar) delivers the hydration of an intense cream with a glorious 'I've just been on holiday' tint; something we all need, because black skin can, and does, go lifeless. The flecks of shimmer might not be everyone's cup of tea but they are subtle and understated, rather than a glitter-fest, and make skin look so much healthier. I must however manage your expectations here: there's a mini-ad that was created to promote Body Lava, where Rihanna's body basically glows like a furnace. This body luminizer is stupendous and will give you a radiant glow, but unless you buy enough product to fill your bathtub and marinate in it for days, please don't expect to look the same. Just saying.

PAULA'S CHOICE
Skin Revealing Body Lotion 10% AHA

In my opinion, traditional body exfoliators are messy, inefficient and a colossal waste of money. My daily body exfoliation routine consists of an 'African sponge' (in reality a piece of mesh) that costs me no more than a pound and does a much better job than its overpriced, grainy comrades. I do, however, make an exception for this. It calls itself a lotion but, technically, it's a non-grainy body-smoothing creamy exfoliator that gets rid of dead skin cells, targets brown spots and treats keratosis pilaris – those non-threatening but nonetheless offensive 'chicken skin' bumps. The benefits don't end there. You don't have to rinse it off which avoids the tiresome mess that is a mainstay of a traditional exfoliator, and its brilliant formulation, which includes much-loved emollient shea butter, green tea and anti-ageing glycolic acid, dissolves those pesky lacklustre skin cells and leaves your skin feeling smooth. To get the best out of this exfoliator, approach it exactly as you would any other acid: slowly. Use it once a week at first, to avoid irritation, and build up from there. Do also bear in mind that whilst it does hydrate your skin, the finish is matte, which might be disappointing if you thrive on a bit of body shine, so use it at night instead and be grateful your sheets don't get greasy. Finally, remember that when you use acids, your skin becomes more susceptible to sun damage so you will need to apply sunscreen on your body. I know, I know, it's a pain. But I promise, it's worth it.

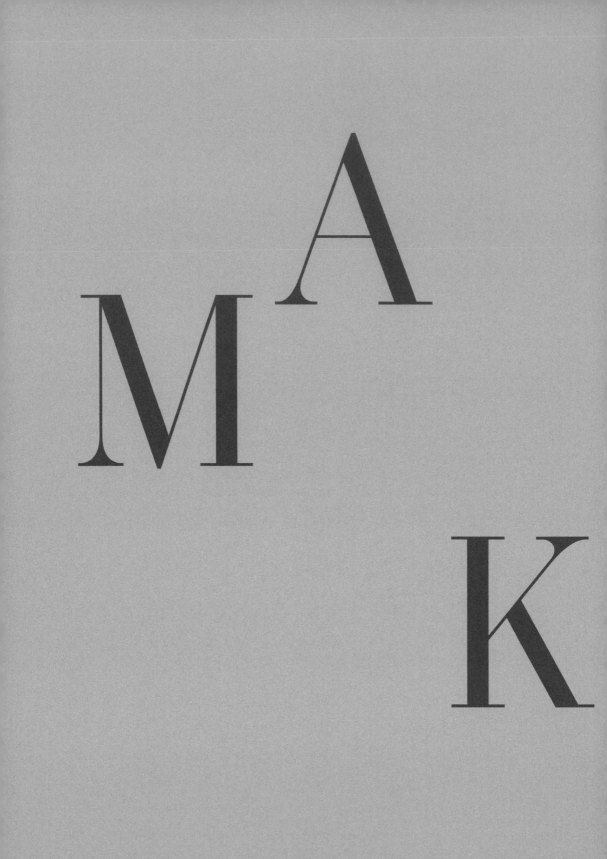

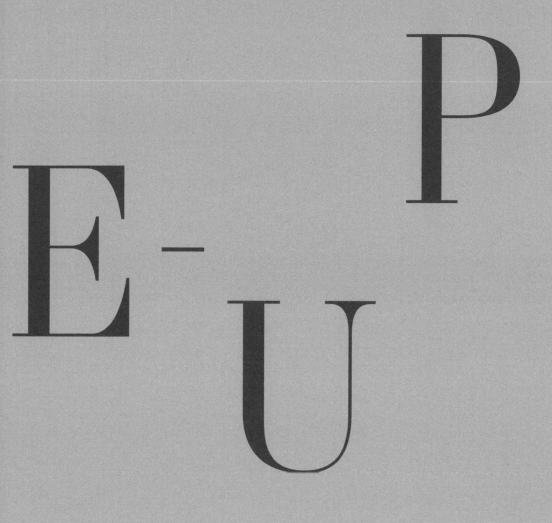

COSMETICS

How much make-up does a girl really need? Does anyone actually need yellow eyeshadow? Can highlighters that make you look like Tin Man ever justify their existence? Will brands ever stop creating those darned matte lipsticks that make your lips feel so brittle they might as well have been marinated in crushed concrete? Needless to say, there is a lot of terrible stuff out there. Conversely, there is also a lot of good stuff.

When I decided to write this book with the idea of featuring beauty products that work brilliantly for women of colour, I told a Caucasian friend of mine who works in the beauty industry. Her response was, 'Where are you going to find it all? Surely the issue is that there is nothing out there?' This seems to be the prevalent viewpoint concerning make-up for women of colour, but I don't agree. There are a lot of great products on the market. You just have to know what they are. In 2017, when Rihanna launched Fenty Beauty, her game-changing, all-inclusive beauty brand, it totally altered the conversation around the issue of inclusivity. More significantly, it made so much money that everyone woke up to the fact that the demographic they had ignored for so long spent a lot on beauty. (Ah, sorry, did I just burst a bubble? Did you really think the industry suddenly felt guilty at their lack of inclusivity and decided to make a positive change for the betterment of society? I wish I were less cynical, but, fundamentally, as with any business, it was a money decision.) If brands such as MAC and Bobbi Brown opened doors, Fenty Beauty essentially came along and kicked those doors off their hinges. Don't get me wrong, it's a work in progress: many foundations still leave you looking like a cantaloupe. Tons of blushers and eyeshadows have yet to be created with pigments deep enough for darker skins. The bulk of lipsticks ignore the fact that many women of colour have naturally dark lips. The numerous brow products supposedly great for dark brows and therefore people of colour are, in reality, only acceptable if you think brows dusted with cigarette ash is a good look. But more than ever before, there are brilliant options available. So, I ask again, how much make-up does a girl really need?

Well, you need at least two great foundations to accommodate the changing seasons. Your choice of lipstick shades will vary as per your mood and event. Navy-blue glittery eyeshadow can be a wonderful thing (trust me on this one) but is probably not Monday-morning boardroom fare, and super glossy lip gloss will celebrate the fullness of our lips, but on a sandy, breezy beach it will never end well. The answer is, we need a lot of make-up, because context is everything. Also think about it this way: discovering and rediscovering make-up products will increase the likelihood of you staying box fresh.

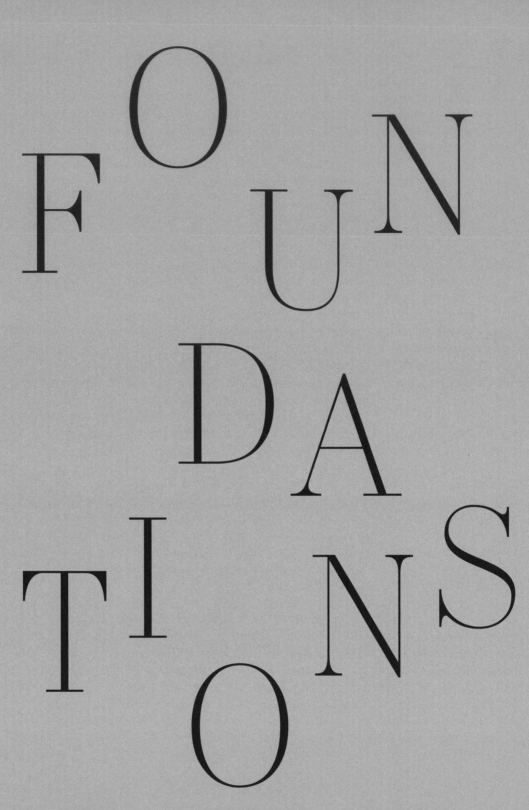

FOUNDATIONS

THINGS TO NOTE...

A foundation is like a bra: most women
are wearing the wrong one, and like
a bra you need a wardrobe of them for
different occasions. For the best 'fit' you
should ideally choose your foundation
in real life rather than digitally; if you
look grey, red or cantaloupe, it is not
the light. Finally, remember, foundation
should complement your skin and
not act as an opaque cover up: it's a
complexion, not a scandal.

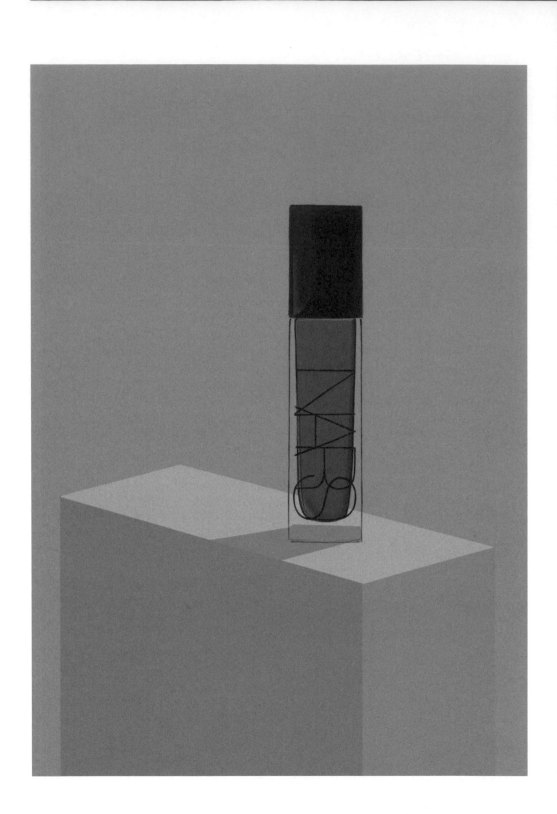

NARS
Natural Radiant Longwear Foundation

I have had a lifelong battle with skin you could fry an egg on, and everyone always tries to make me feel better about it by saying, 'Ah, but just think, you'll look so young when you're 80.' I mean, at that point, who gives a monkey's? Anyway, needless to say, I have always admired and coveted a supremely matte face. Problem is, it doesn't love me back. A totally matte face makes me look as if I've had a sense-of-humour failure. On days when I have nothing more pressing to think about, I consider my ideal-scenario foundation. Well, first, it needs to be the right colour, otherwise I may as well just go back to bed. Second, the texture should be not quite matte, not shiny but something in between (a finish we now know as 'dewy'). Additionally, it must cover niggling pigmentation issues and have more longevity than the career of an *X Factor* winner, and it shouldn't oxidise quicker than a cheap apple or leave a mark on everyone and everything in sight.

That is the dream, and this comes pretty close. It is a beautifully blurring, modern concoction that comes with added skincare benefits – raspberry, apple and watermelon extracts to improve skin texture over time. It gets top marks for giving you that 'Have you been away?' luminosity. It also stays put all day, which should be standard. If you have a foundation that constantly needs reapplying because it is slipping and sliding like a drunk with vertigo, you need to kick it to the curb. Non-foundation wearers are always terrified to foray into foundations because they have a preconceived idea that they have the texture of batter and feel uncomfortable. They are not far off the mark: many do. This one, on the other hand, is lightweight, natural looking (yes, even at full coverage) and totally buildable. It comes in thirty-five shades, which is great. However, let's not get too caught up in shade ranges. I applaud beauty brands going beyond the norm, but let's keep it in context. A 100-shade range of foundations sounds impressive, but if the formulation is a shocker, all you have is a bad foundation in 100 shades. This, of course, is the opposite. It is brilliant but not so brilliant that it won't transfer on to your white shirt if you're not careful. Just keeping it real.

DIOR
Forever Skin Glow

One of the biggest issues any foundation-wearer faces – aside from that small, unimportant thing of not being able to find the right colour – is finding a non-matte foundation that goes the distance. It is a tricky Holy Grail formulation to get right. Dior is one of the small number of brands that has managed to achieve this. Their cult-classic Dior Forever has been reformulated into a long-wear 24-hour formula, and it is available in two finishes, matte and glow. Both have impressive skincare benefits: pansy extract as a hydration booster, rose hip extract to refine skin texture and pores, and SPF35 to protect skin from environmental aggressors. The sunscreen is a clever addition for those who deem sun protection as tedious as ironing. My personal go-to is the glow. The pigment is intense, which means you don't need much to get full coverage; the (flawless) finish, however, is natural looking. It has been created for drier skin types, but if you are oily and want a little bit of a glow without looking like you've just swum in a pool of crude oil, this is a safe bet. A few things worth noting: when choosing your shade, the trite adage 'don't judge a book by its cover' really applies. You cannot pick your shade simply by looking at the colour in the bottle because it blends into skin in a way that is unexpected. In a moment of boredom, I tried one that looked practically orange. It was crazy watching it blend seamlessly into my skin; I would have never automatically chosen it. Trying to buy this online might be a challenge; like attempting a conversation via Google Translate, it will, inevitably, result in confusion.

BECCA
Ultimate Coverage
24 Hour Foundation

It's funny how we find happiness in the most unlikely places. Who knew that a make-up brand created in Australia, by a white Australian woman, would be so ahead of its time in the area of inclusivity and bring me – and thousands of other women – so much joy? This is not one of the brands that hit the market with a whitewashed range of foundations and justifying it with the inane excuse 'we just want to see how these go first'. Every time I hear this, I am baffled. How does the commercial success of foundations for whiter skin tones relate to the decision (or not) to cater for darker skin tones? Or have I missed something here? Another excuse is 'Well, it's expensive to launch a wide range'. Both completely valid reasons to discount an entire demographic. The fact BECCA went against the grain impressed me. At that point it was what you might describe as a niche brand, but its foundation shade range was extensive – super pale to really deep – and its campaigns featured women of colour. This was all at a time no one was talking about inclusivity; yet, for BECCA, it wasn't even a thing, it was the norm. For me, though, it was a big deal and I have since recommended it to friends and family members who are white, black, mixed, and every shade in between and they have all become enamoured with it too. And here's why: it provides, as it says, the 'ultimate coverage'; coverage so impressive your acne scarring doesn't stand a chance. Equally, if you mix it with **Shimmering Skin Perfector® Liquid Highlighter**, everyone will covet your skin: it's that incredible. The consistency is a thick, creamy paste, of which, unless you have an exceptionally big face, you don't need very much: two pumps should do the trick. The shade range is extensive, although it could do with a few in-betweeners; if you struggle, consider buying two shades next to each other and playing alchemist. No, not ideal, but it is worth it, because this not-quite-matte, not-quite-dewy hybrid is skin perfection in a bottle.

LANCÔME
Le Teint Particulier
Custom Made Foundation

The opportunity to have my make-up done is a regular part of the job. But I really don't like it. Other beauty editors relish the idea of being made up by some of the world's most lauded make-up artists, but it fills me with horror. I don't want my skin scrutinised. It's akin to when you see your dentist, and she tuts as if she's never seen a cavity before. On occasions when I've gone against my better judgement and allowed myself to be made up, I look in the mirror and either think, I could have done a better job myself, or, who the hell is that?! Also, unless I'm having a facial, I don't like my face being touched (it's bacteria fear – never mind Don't Touch My Hair; Don't Touch My Face). And then this came up. How could I hold out on a personalised foundation with the potential to develop a mind-boggling 70,000+ hues?

The experience was unexpectedly straightforward – and fascinating. A device, a cross between an old-school mobile phone and a remote control – is scanned over your face to detect your (varying) skin tone. You then answer a series of questions about your skin type, coverage required and so on. This information goes into the system, and then the magic begins. A machine plops the various percentages of colours (all dependent on your skin tone and undertone) into a see-through tube. This combination is whirred up in what looks like the spinning function of a washing machine and, boom, you have your very own personal foundation. It is then packaged up in a chic bottle and box with your name and 'complexion ID', which is handy for reordering. The whole process took around twenty minutes, and the colour was spot on. The formula was oil and fragrance free, perfect for full coverage, and proved to be long-wearing, while the finish, a radiant dewiness, gave me the best version of my skin. Still, the cliché 'you get what you put into it' is apt here. The machine thinks oily skins automatically want a matte foundation; if you tick 'oily skin' on the earlier questionnaire, you will get a matte foundation. For something less matte tick 'normal'. So, yes, this is not without its flaws, but let's be honest, it could be worse – I could have ended up with a foundation that makes me look grey. The two things I can imagine (and understand) people complaining about, however, regard accessibility. First, this service is not currently widely available. I went to Harrods on a Monday morning, which was serene; (a weekend foray into this busy Knightsbridge store is anxiety inducing). The second issue is the price. It is at least two to three times more expensive than an off-the-peg foundation. However, if you've searched high and low, and still have trouble finding a foundation to your liking, consider it a worthy investment.

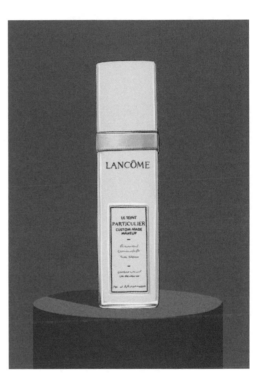

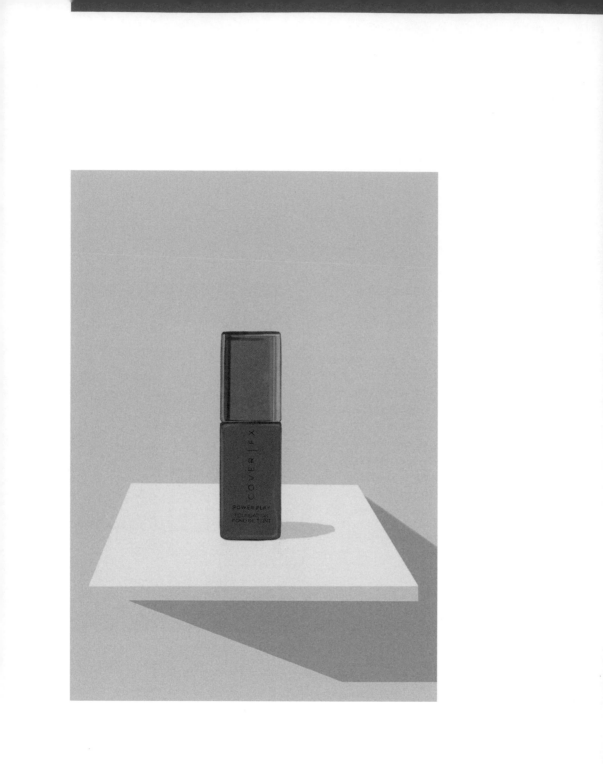

COVER FX
Power Play Foundation

By complete accident, I wore a Cover FX foundation on my wedding day. A week before, I was on my way to interview the formulator behind the then little-known brand when my phone rang. My bridal make-up artist was pulling out due to unforeseen circumstances. Long story short, one of the Cover FX team, a fellow woman of colour, stepped in and ended up as my make-up artist. Consequently, I have always had a soft spot for Cover FX, but if you had told me then that it would become a sexy, Insta-famous brand, I would have laughed in your face. It wasn't cool, it wasn't coveted, and the packaging was a horror. But the formulations were good, and this incarnation is even more impressive. The putty-like substance provides an incredible coverage that is blurred and non-cakey. It is a matte finish but not so matte you look dead inside. If you want what I sometimes refer to as a 'juicy' finish, then I would suggest blending it with a liquid highlighter. Alternatively, you could add either a few drops of hyaluronic acid for an extra boost of moisture or another lighter but more dewy foundation. Once the foundation has been applied it will not budge, which, in one sense, is great (no one wants a moving-target foundation); in another sense it is annoying, given that malleability and blendability, to my mind, are the pillars of a good foundation. The packaging is also all at once genius and exasperating. I love that stumpy but modern rectangular shape that is easy to travel with. The nozzle is great for getting the product out: the difference between tomato ketchup in a glass bottle and its squeezy relative. However, when the bottle is less full, getting the stuff out is like trying to coax a child out of a sweet shop. Ultimately, there are a lot of positives, such as the ease with which you can find your shade (there are forty, with varied undertones) via the clever online guide. Alas, not all stockists carry all the shades. But let's not even get started on that one.

YSL
Touche Eclat Le Teint/All-In-One Glow/All Hours Liquid

There are three foundations from one brand here, and I'll explain why. My choice of foundation depends on what my face is doing and on what I'm doing. There have been times (particularly while writing this book) when I realise I haven't been outside for days. On day five, I suddenly remember I have an important beauty-industry event, at which a camera is never far away, and then I look in the mirror and see a decomposing corpse staring back at me. On such days, my face requires three foundations and a highlighter. For the days when I am not doing anything special, I will slap on a little low-maintenance foundation, so I don't frighten people on public transport. It is just good manners, really.

Whatever my foundation requirements, I find something from YSL always makes the cut. Touche Éclat Le Teint is one of the rare foundations that I actually finish. It is their best-seller, and when you use it, you'll understand why. This full-coverage base (with an incredible 'glow') feels and applies like a serum, which is especially perfect for the days you don't have the energy to do anything with precision. It also works as a great 'off-duty' foundation – for when you

want to look decent but not too 'done'. If you sometimes suffer from that modern-day malady, raging insomnia, and have a face that shows it, adorn yourself with this, and no one would ever guess. It is amazing. It blends beautifully with liquid and powder highlighters, doesn't pill over primer, and even though it covers a multitude of sins, it still gives a human-like finish. Yet nothing is perfect; if you have incredibly oily skin, keep blotting powder to hand so you don't end up looking like an oil rig. The shades are still not as extensive as they could be, so there is a limit to finding your exact match. For those who can, though, it's a beauty.

Now if you want all the benefits of Le Teint with a lighter finish, All-In-One Glow is hydrating, oil free, super dewy and less opaque. The nifty, squeezy 30ml packaging makes it brilliant for travelling, and if you like to wear make-up on holiday, this will help you avoid that 'overdone reality-TV star' look.

All Hours does exactly what it says on the tin – it lasts for 24 hours. Now, of course, if you were to wear your foundation for

24 hours, I'd wager that something had gone horribly wrong. However, the point is that this is an 'on the dance floor all night' kind of foundation; 'she works hard for the money' and all that. The high-pigment formula is waterproof and non-transferable – up to a point (it's not as if it dries like ink; let's be realistic here). Oilier skin tones with a penchant for a matte finish will love it; dry skin tones may find it better to stick to the aforementioned two. What's the final thing that sets all these apart from other foundations? They smell wonderful. So, if anyone gets really close, they may want to spend all day sniffing your face. Just so you know.

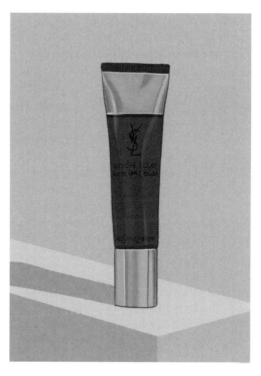

HUDA BEAUTY
#FauxFilter Foundation

For those who covet that HD-perfect, 'more is more', Instagram-pervasive skin that makes you look like you've swallowed Facetune, this foundation is a requisite. I am aware that this kind of look comes under fire for not reflecting reality or a 'natural' beauty, and, no, it is not my beauty school of thought. (I applaud your tenacity and patience in creating this face daily; I have no idea where you find the energy.) But, whatever; if you fall into this camp, there's no shame in it. One of the things I love about beauty is the democracy of it all. Wear it how you like it.

As the name on the bottle suggests, this is the sort of foundation with a flawlessness akin to a filter (fitting, as founder Huda Kattan built her eponymous billion-dollar brand via social media). While #FauxFilter may sound like marketing hyperbole, the point is that when it says full coverage, it means business. If you are a minimalist kind of girl, whose idea of a full face of make-up is lip gloss, mascara and tinted moisturiser, this is your nemesis. The brand alludes to the coverage level being adjustable, but let's just call a spade a spade: it's a full-coverage foundation.

So, barely there girls should look elsewhere and foundation maximalists, read on.

You don't need much of this foundation to get that blurring–flawless effect; any more than a couple of pumps (tops), and the result is 'more is more is more' madness. This finish is totally matte and incredibly long wearing; when used in conjunction with a primer and a decent finishing powder, your foundation will be everything-proof. This is wonderful news for oilier skins. However, while some hydrating-boosting ingredients – argan oil and centella asiatica – have been added to the formulation, this foundation dries to a powdery, velvety finish. Some drier skins might struggle with this, and I have heard complaints that it settles into the cracks. Still there are key elements that endear me to this product: Huda Kattan's personal experience with problematic skin inspired her to develop a formulation that also works for acne suffers, something to which most foundations cannot lay claim. Her 30-strong selection (which incorporates a range of undertones) has been developed to cater to those who have traditionally been marginalised by the beauty industry. For that alone, it's a winner.

GIORGIO ARMANI
Power Fabric/ Luminous Silk

The problem with a brand creating completely different products in almost identical packaging is that, invariably, there will be a case of mistaken identity. I can remember trying an Armani foundation many years back and not loving it, but then not remembering exactly which one it was. This is what deterred me for so long from retrying a foundation from the brand. And then I worked with someone whose make-up always looked so dreamy. What foundation does she use? Giorgio Armani. And so here we are.

Let's start with Power Fabric. This has made numerous 'ultimate oily skin foundation' awards, but if you were to (ill) judge it on the texture alone, you would say those lists were rigged (many are, to be honest). It is thick, luxe, creamy, luminous and full coverage with added sun protection (SPF25), everything, indeed, that indicates it would crank up your oil supply and break you out. But it doesn't. In fact, on application, this astute formulation goes on like a silky, matte second skin. As with most mattes, it is also very long wearing (drier skins, hydrate first, so you don't crack under the pressure); normal skins will also love it. If, ultimately, you just don't like a matte foundation then there's no point trying to fit a square peg in a round hole.

If you are looking for a true lightweight, then you are better off going for Luminous Silk. The clue is in the name: it gives you that slightly blurred, luminous finish normally only achievable with lights, cameras and Instagram filters. It is also super silky on the skin but not overly dewy; if you want a little more glow, you will need to add a few drops of a highlighter or hydrator. Now it says it is buildable, but let's keep it real: it won't build to the point where it covers everything. If you prefer a full-coverage foundation, your reaction may well be 'Who let the tinted moisturiser in?'. Those with a predilection for less is more, however, will be utterly delighted.

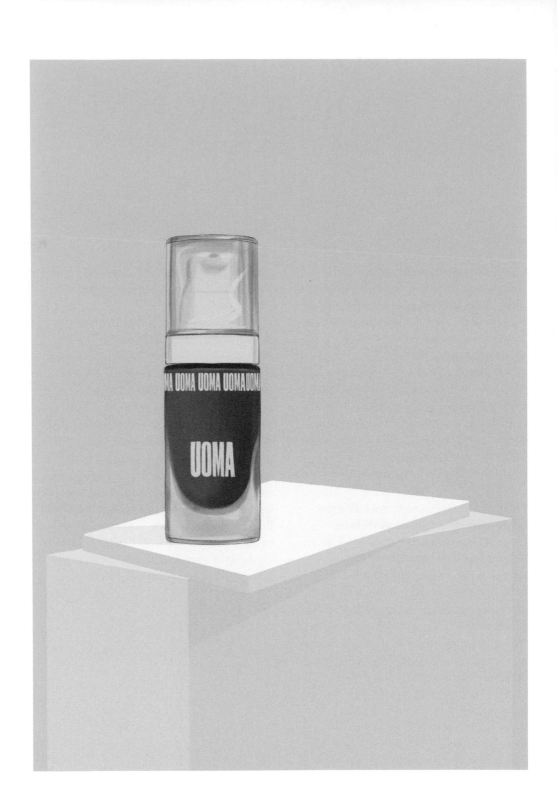

UOMA BEAUTY
Say What?! Foundation

When I met Sharon Chuter, the Nigerian-born Australian founder of UOMA, we had a long, impassioned conversation about the issues you face as a woman of colour in the industry. When she showed me the products that she planned to launch to address these issues, I was blown away. The thinking behind the brand is nothing short of genius: it is a celebration of Africa and its diaspora that also invites people outside of the demographic to 'join the tribe'. This foundation is the star of the collection. Its all-inclusive range caters to 51 different skin shades, taking undertones into consideration – you may need to try a few to get the right shade – but it's the formulation that makes it a standout.

Using the Fitzpatrick scale which measures the skin's reaction to the sun, UOMA has identified six 'skin kins' that everyone falls into: White Pearl, Fair Lady, Honey Honey, Bronze Venus, Brown Sugar and Black Pearl. Each foundation includes ingredients to cater to their kin's needs, such as brightening tomato extract to counteract Black Pearl's tendency towards dullness. All the foundations also include a 'biomimicry' pigment to match the skin tone but blur it, meaning the look of pores and lines are minimised. Thanks to the injection of hyaluronic acid, the matte end result is fresh and velvety rather than one that makes you look lifeless. Now that's what I call a good foundation.

Keep moistu
serums, foun
nail varnishe
fridge. They
a longer shel
on like a dre

sers,
ations and
in the
ill have
ife and go
n.

KEVYN AUCOIN
The Sensual Skin Enhancer Concealer

When this product first came out, I had no idea what it was. Thankfully, there was no need to hide my ignorance for fear of looking like a fool – no one else had a clue what it was either. All we knew was that it made your skin look epic. My shade in this small, round pot of intense pigment looks a bit like a chocolate ganache. It is thick, like a heavy paste, which is, initially, perturbing; when it goes on your skin the results are quite stunning.

So how does one use it? Well, as a concealer, it will cover a multitude of afflictions. As a highlighter – just pick one or two shades lighter – it will help your face catch the light in the most natural way (it's an enhancer, remember?). It won't shimmer like the glow-in-the-dark meets Tin Man homage that everyone seems to (over)indulge in these days. However, if you decide to use this as a foundation, there are some things you should know. Yes, it will give you the most divine blurred-velvety-dewy finish. Yes, you will benefit from the infusion of honey and jojoba oil. Yes, it will give you maximum coverage, but go easy. 'Use sparingly' should be at the forefront of your mind – go overboard, and you will look like you're wearing a balaclava. It is that intense. Use it correctly, and it

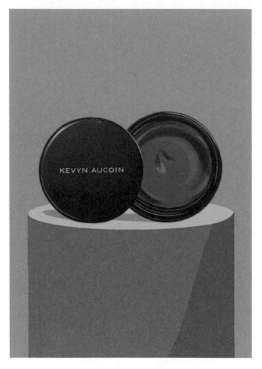

will look and feel like skin. If you find the texture too dense or not pliable enough, I recommend (for all skin types) mixing in a liquid highlighter or an incredibly hydrating serum, which will help it glide on more smoothly, while giving you coverage without the heaviness. The only downside is that it smells like an expensive smoky chocolate. I struggle with gourmand beauty, but if you must smell like chocolate, just please make it Dairy Milk.

ESTEE LAUDER
Double Wear Stay-in-Place Makeup SPF 10

This is the UK's best-selling foundation, apparently. It has such cult status that no one even refers to it by its full name or brand any more. It's just known as Double Wear. I've long been aware of it, of course – it is quite old school – but I was late to the party. While I am promiscuous with my choice of lipsticks (give me a good non-drying liquid matte, and I'm all yours), I take a little more wooing when it comes to swapping one of the six foundations I have in rotation at any given time. Yes, I know that sounds excessive, and yes, it is somewhat sacrilegious for a beauty editor never to have tried the best-selling foundation in the country, so of course I had to give in, and I'm so glad I did. It is a gloopy, glossy beauty with the texture of melted chocolate. The coverage is buildable but not full; if you are a full-coverage kind of girl, see this as your base for dress-down days. It has been, quite rightly, applauded for its extensive shade range (60+) and for the fact that it is utterly immovable: resistant to heat, humidity and perspiration (because that always sounds less offensive than sweat). The downside with this USP is that once it hits your skin, it is not the easiest of products to move around. They do say it is non-transferable, and it sort of is and isn't. If you have drier, fairer skin then it is less likely to come off on your clothes. If you are darker skinned or have oily skin and decide to wear a cream silk dress, well, it's a little more complicated.

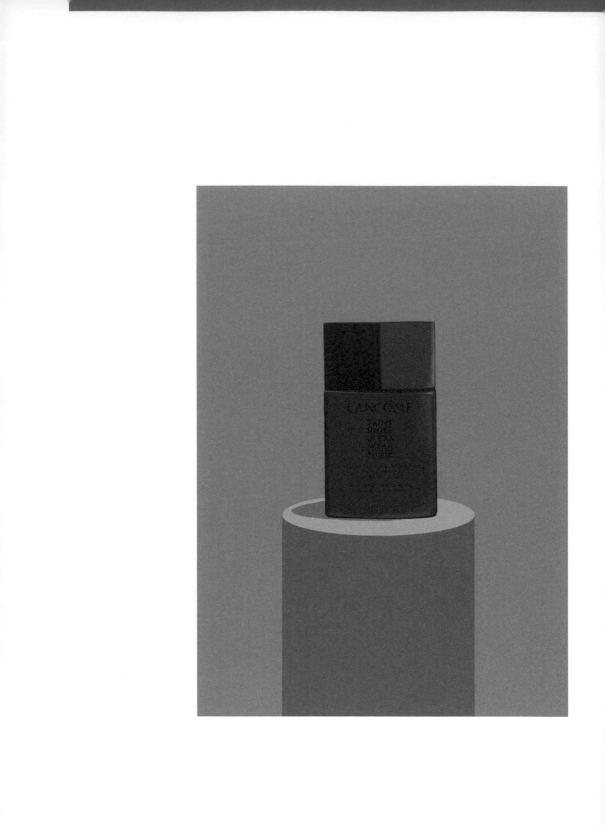

LANCÔME
Teint Idole
Ultra Wear Nude

After years of being tortured by the word nude – nude tights, nude lipstick, nude bras – denoting a colour that does not resemble my skin tone, I find the word jarring. However, using it to describe a range of foundations that suits numerous skin tones – that is, every type of 'nude' makes complete sense. Lancôme's classic Teint Idole Ultra Wear is the brand's brilliant and continually improved long-lasting full-coverage formula. Think of 'Nude' as its sexier, lighter-coverage twin. The consistency is perfect for a no-make-up make-up look that has enough substance to convince people you haven't simply dragged yourself out of the house without looking in the mirror. If you want much more coverage, you'd be better off trying a full-coverage foundation rather than trying to layer this and ending up like a badly assembled lasagne. Beyond its coverage, it smells amazing, like a floral-scented skincare product – not something the anti-fragrance brigade would be happy with, but there you go. It comes in forty shades, which are balanced: no tagging on the darker shades like unexpected (and uninvited) guests. In order to ensure it has the right consistency, you must shake the bottle before use. Once on, it is beautiful: a silky pigment-rich, incredibly lightweight, skin-like base. Just before this launched, I met Balanda Atis, the awesome woman-of-colour scientist behind the incredible formulations at Lancôme. Something of a superstar in beauty circles, she has made it her mission to ensure that every woman, everywhere, can find her own nude. For that alone, I love this foundation.

ILLAMASQUA
Skin Base Foundation

Unbeknown to a lot of my friends and family, they are my guinea pigs. I don't think that is a terrible thing. I am sent a million-and-one beauty products, and unless I grow ten heads and spend every waking hour faffing around with them, there is no way I could use or try everything for any length of time. Years ago, I sent this foundation to a friend as I was not quite ready to road test it. A few months down the line I had a frantic call from her saying she had run out and couldn't get her shade. She is a tough customer, so this was good news for what turned out to be a brilliant foundation.

There is a part of me that loves the packaging. It is wonderfully dinky and easy to cart around (transportable, as I once heard someone say, which still doesn't register as a proper word, but it's in the dictionary, so there you go). Brands assume that you never want to travel with your foundation but, you know, sometimes you do and the less cumbersome it is, the better. Saying all that, there is another side of me that doesn't like the packaging at all: the squeezy tube gets irritatingly inefficient as it begins to empty. You would end up either wasting tons of product or cutting it open with a serrated knife. Neither holds appeal. Now, per ml, it sounds pricey, but you need so little of it on a daily basis, it will prove excellent value for money. Illamasqua says this provides the ultimate skin-realism effect. And this is true. It does look like your skin, well, its airbrushed, red-carpet-walking alter ego anyway. The texture is thick – which is just as well, or it would go everywhere – it is easily blendable and doesn't oxidise. The game changer for me, however, is that you can purchase sample pots via the Illamasqua website. This means the risk of getting stuck with a full bottle of foundation that makes you look like a completely different person is greatly diminished.

LAURA MERCIER
Flawless Lumiēre Radiance-Perfecting Foundation

It might not be a sexy-millennial Insta-famous brand, but Laura Mercier has been at the forefront of the flawless face for years. And, judging by this foundation, LM could still run rings around its upstart counterparts. If super matte and super dewy had a love child, this would be it: perfect for those who love the **Flawless Fusion Ultra-Longwear Foundation** but find it just that little bit too matte. This, on the other hand, is magnificently creamy; the sort of finish that makes you stare narcissistically at yourself in the mirror. The pigment is deep and evens out the skin – yes, even scarring, blemishes and so forth – with the tiniest amount, but it's not just about covering up, it also corrects. The injection of vitamin C means illumination is all yours. I don't mean the highlighting sort, I mean the sort that over time, reduces the intensity of your dark spots and gives you an off-the-scale radiance. Finally, there's your 15-hour intense boost of hydration, which is all thanks to the silver ear mushroom. No, I didn't know this existed either, but seeing as it stops your face from turning into a prune, I think we should just say thank you; no questions asked.

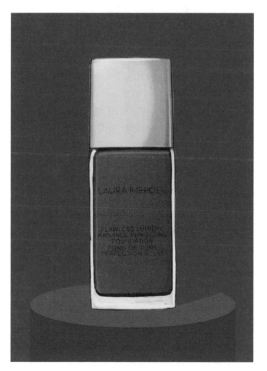

FENTY BEAUTY
Pro Filt'r Soft Matte Longwear Foundation

If you haven't heard of this then you have probably been living under a rock. The launch of the 40-strong shade range was the catalyst that drove the narrative around increased inclusivity in the beauty industry. Beauty brands are now placing the issue of representation at the forefront of their strategy, and it's all down to Rihanna. Of course, there are still high-profile beauty products launching that may as well be named 'no people of colour allowed'. However, the progress being made is the most exciting and forward-looking change that has taken place in decades. Pro Filt'r is the foundation I have been asked about the most, so it was important to include it in the book. With all the hype and the coverage (pun very much intended) you'd expect this to be the most incredible foundation you have ever used in your life. That is too high an expectation.

With that in mind, here's what everyone needs to know. The foundation is quite liquidy, which can be problematic if you are overly zealous with the pump. However, there are pros to this texture: it is lightweight and easy to apply. The finish is a beautiful modern matte – that is, not the kind that makes you look as if you forgot to moisturise. If, however, you prefer a dewy finish, this is not ideal. And if your skin is dry, it's worth using a few drops of a hyaluronic acid and a hydrating primer before applying the foundation – wait for it to dry before layering it, otherwise it will pill. Coverage wise it is medium but buildable, to which I often think, who has time to put on another two layers every morning? For a lightweight matte, blurring finish, however, it's perfect.

There are things to keep in mind: colours that automatically look like your shade could be wrong; the subtle but significant difference is all in the undertone. Some red, some yellow… but next to each other, they look fairly identical. If you are not able to get to a counter, the Fenty Beauty website has a pretty good guide for choosing foundation shades. If you are wavering between two, you're advised always to go for the lighter, as the dry-down will be darker. This is a concept I find slightly alarming. Your dry-down could leave you with the perfect colour (which is what it is supposed to do). But there is also a chance that you end up with an 'oxidisation on speed' face. So get your shade right and you'll have a silky matte, perfectly blurred Fenty face.

BY TERRY
Terrybly Densiliss® Foundation

I don't tend to use the word luxurious these days as its meaning has become ambiguous and is open to interpretation – a bit like the terms 'iconic' or 'influencer'. But I have to contradict myself and say: this is a luxurious foundation. Yes, you could argue that the beautiful, rich and clever formulation (and the price) falls firmly under 'luxury', but it is more than that. It is an almost indefinable thing, but when you see luxury, you know it. I'll admit, the shade range isn't huge, but if you can find yours here, it is worth exploring, particularly if you have more mature skin. Most brands do not consider how their foundations will sit on older skins – perhaps they imagine everyone is Peter Pan, and ageing is some life-threatening disease we should all hope to never get?

This, on the other hand, has been created with the older woman in mind; yet works beautifully on everyone. It is a skincare–make-up hybrid that corrects and perfects (one ingredient, a mimetic factor, boosts collagen levels, whilst a flawless time-control complex smooths out lines), and leaves your skin looking radiant, blurred and polished. Something to note: this serum-like foundation is intensely pigmented, so avoid applying without a brush. Use your fingers, and your tips will look as if you have been at the police station having your prints taken. (I haven't experienced this myself; I've just watched a lot of *Law & Order*.) The stain is testament to the strength of the pigment; it is bothersome, and you do have to wash your hands to get it off properly. It is a small price to pay, though, for a foundation that glides on like silk and doesn't languish in your creases. I should rephrase that: there is nothing 'small price' about this foundation. But, in this case, you get what you pay for.

CONCEAL-ERS & CORRECT-ORS

THINGS TO NOTE...

Brightener-concealers (the best kind) are exactly that. They should brighten, and they should conceal. But not to the point where either you glow in the dark or no one can find you. Discover a good one, and it will cover dark circles, distract from blemishes and make you look a million times more youthful. Don't leave home without it.

MAC
Studio Finish SPF 35 Concealer

This is the first concealer I ever used and fell in love with. To me it was and still is a little pot of magic. Most concealers have imposter syndrome; rightly so. They have no idea who they are or what they are doing. Some are too thin to make a difference. Others leave a greasy coat; still others are so dry you might as well have crushed cement under your eyes. Then, of course, there is the flimsy inconsistent texture that doesn't conceal anything. I mean, what's the point of that? Most concealers these days are radiant fluids, which is wonderfully modern, and they have their upsides and their place. However, if you are looking for a properly matte finish (something so many concealers lack) that still maintains a certain level of moisture (not greasiness; there's a difference) then this is a terrific option that has much going for it. It is brightening, filled with antioxidants, water resistant, fragrance free and 'non-acnegenic' (MAC's word; not mine), which means that if you have acne, it won't make it worse. The texture is a cross between filler and pâté; you don't need much, so it lasts an age. I remember having a particular one for years, but unless you thrive on recurring conjunctivitis, I wouldn't recommend holding on to it for that long. The pot is great value for money so you will literally be able to get every little morsel out of it (use a brush though, to avoid the spread of germs). And I would store it out of sunlight and, ideally, keep it in the fridge – it is much more effective that way and stays wonderfully opaque. This, to some, might sound nightmarish, but for anyone with dark circles, pigmentation and an uneven skin tone, it is a weightless, brightening dream of a thing. The best concealers should blend but not disappear into your foundation, which this doesn't; nevertheless you should apply it pre foundation, particularly around the eye area. Which reminds me: am I the only one who thinks we have taken concealer abuse to another level? For everyone still sporting reverse panda eyes as some kind of badge of honour, please, take it down a notch.

NARS
Radiant Creamy Concealer

I love going to a NARS launch. It is one where I know I won't have someone passing me something with more peach tones than the *FT* while saying, 'Yes, I know it's not quite your colour (aka I'm so woke I recognise that) but just thought you could try it for texture?' Sorry, I know I am being harsh but it just gets a little Groundhog Day. At NARS there is always something for everyone. I recall this launching and being so utterly thrilled at the range of colours available. I am told it is the number-one selling concealer in the US; all the beauty editors love it, and it has a loyal cult following. And it's obvious why – it is super creamy so won't drag across your skin (as if you need any more problems). It is infused with lots of skincare benefits – it is incredibly hydrating – and it also leaves a radiant, brightening finish. It is wonderfully non-comedogenic, so it won't clog your pores. It is medium weight, so if you are prone to breakouts and need heavy coverage, this might not hit the spot – quite literally. If you are in the market for something matte, again, look elsewhere –

the clue is in the name. For more mature or dry skins, however, this is brilliant. It will not suck the moisture out of your skin or get stuck in your creases; it will give you a softer, smoother complexion and, shock horror, you'll actually be able to get it in your own colour.

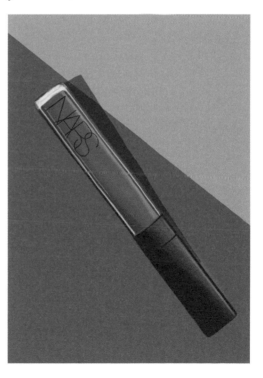

MAYBELLINE
Instant Anti-Age
Eraser Eye Concealer

Is this a safe space? I am hoping it is, hence, I'll admit that I can be a little bit of a snob when it comes to mass, mainstream brands. I say this because I do find, more times than not, the quality (from packaging to content) to be wanting. And I do like things to look nice: being cheap is one thing; looking cheap another. That said, I know it is important not to have a blanket approach, otherwise you miss out on goodies like this. Now let's not gloss over it – there is nothing luxe about this. It is a totally mass-market, inoffensive, forgettable-looking thing. But it's the stuff inside that counts. This brilliant value-for-money concealer is medium-to-high coverage, blends easily into skin and gives you a freshness that hides the fact you are up at night thinking, where on earth is my life going? It is hydrating but, conversely, leaves a powdery finish. When I say this I don't mean that bleak-looking finish that is totally devoid of life. I mean powdery in the sense that it is a hydrated matte that also makes the skin look fresher and smoother, which is what your under eye needs when the reality of your life is giving you dark circles the size of saucers. If there is any concern it is the sponge (which is also a USP). It is a great way to blend the product around the face, but then there's the hygiene issue. The tip is protected with an antimicrobial system; therefore washing it is counterproductive. Your best bet is to clean the tip with a dry tissue every time you use it. Other issues, however, are the availability of shades – thirteen on the last count, with a relatively good balance of dark shades – and that it is quite tricky to find. But if you can get hold of it, do. It offers great coverage, feels like skincare and is reasonably priced. A damn sight better than the plenty of pitiful concealers on the market that are at least three times the price.

BECCA
Aqua Luminous Perfecting Concealer

I have had a relationship with BECCA for a long time, and the honeymoon period is still not over. I bore people with my stories of when we first met; how I discovered one of my favourite foundations and how I am still very much in love. It's like dealing with a smugly-married person. I'm about to do it all again, so forgive me; I apologise in advance. There is still a plethora of make-up with no skincare benefits whatsoever. Considering these are products that will be sitting on your skin all day, that's just daft. This highly pigmented concealer, on the other hand, has been created with skincare in mind. Integrating skin-smoothing ingredients, such as squalane, manuka honey and vitamin E, the silky but sturdy texture applies like a serum. It is immediately brightening – I use it around my eyes and on any dull, uneven parts of my skin, and I swear it's as if someone switched on the lights. This is down to the light-reflecting technology and soft-focus pigments (no, your pores won't completely disappear – sorry! – but they will be blurred). The consistency blends seamlessly into the skin (ideally, apply pre foundation). It comes in a wonderfully inclusive shade range and is highly pigmented, so you don't need very much. It is luminous (not oily – some brands, obviously, can't tell the difference), and doesn't settle in your laughter lines, making you look a million times older. It is also waterproof, which, I suppose, means it's great to take on holiday. Why you'd need to wear concealer while swimming is beyond me but, hey-ho, each to their own. My only teeny criticism is that the application stick doesn't work well in areas where you need a bit more definition, such as around the brows. For that, you'll need a brush. But this is not enough to quench my love for BECCA. Hopefully, nothing will. I expect if they ever did launch a terrible product, I'd take to my bed nursing a broken heart with a huge slice of humble pie.

CHARLOTTE TILBURY
Magic Away Liquid Concealer

This product has been described, in turn, as 'like Spanx for your face', 'your ride-or-die concealer' and 'a magic wand that makes your skin dreams come true'. This is the issue with hype: it is so detrimental to free thinking. And it is near impossible to live up to such (usually unrealistic) expectations. But is this product any good? Well, actually, it's better than good: it's great. Let's talk aesthetics. There is quite a lot of fabulousness going on here.

I have always said that Charlotte Tilbury is clever, because she knows there is a huge coterie of women for whom 'look and feel' make all the difference. To a degree, I am one of those women. Yes, I will always take substance over style, but what's wrong with having both? There is enough ugliness in the world; if a woman gets a kick from a concealer encased in a glamorous rose-gold pen, then all power to her, I say.

The concealer (which took five years to develop and currently features sixteen shades) is creamy, pigment rich and luminous but not overly oily – my biggest issue with most 'hydrating' concealers. It gives great coverage – they say, full, I say, medium but buildable – but it still feels and looks like skin. The ingredients are very much skincare focused: Persian silk tree bark extract, Bliss Molecule (the scientific name is palmitoyal glycine, known to assist in the reduction of lines and wrinkles) and wild indigo to reduce dark circles, wrinkles and crow's feet, as well as blemishes and imperfections. But the pièce de résistance, for me, is the foamy 'magic precision cushion applicator' at the nib of the pen. It is truly genius. You twist the bottom of the pen, the concealer comes through, and you apply it: easy, smoothing, comfortable and luxe. It works like a Beautyblender for your under-eye area and is a million times more practical than the ubiquitous stick applicators. Is it a wand that makes your skin dreams come true? I mean, while I am a bit allergic to that sort of marketing blurb, there is no denying, it is a little bit of magic in a pen.

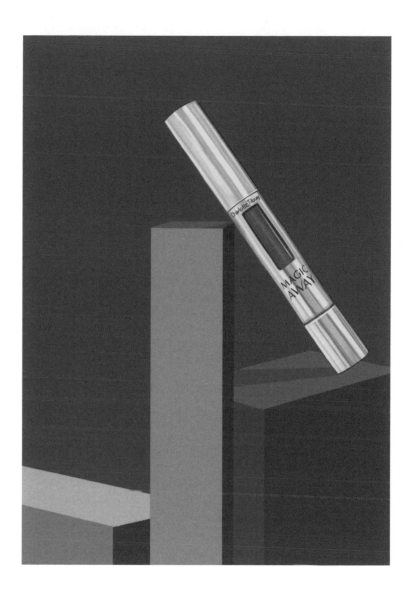

URBAN DECAY
Naked Skin Weightless Complete Coverage Concealer

There are so many concealers that claim to be full coverage, and yet when I try them, I begin to question my capacity to understand English. Note to brands: if I have to layer it a million times in order to cover dark circles everyone can still see, that is not full coverage. This Urban Decay concealer, however, is bang on the money. I generally find products with long names reek of indecision, but, in this case, I will forgive that, because the key to brilliance here is in the name: Naked Skin. Expect this to give you a finish that looks as if you have nothing on. It will look like skin, but the airbrushed version, because that's the point: it's weightless. You won't feel like you have anything on. If you think about it in terms of fabric, it's a lovely expensive silk. This is an important point, because tons of concealers are so heavy that if they were a fabric, they would be corduroy.

Complete Coverage: this is what is so exciting. It manages to cover everything and be pretty much opaque while maintaining all of those naked skin and weightless elements. What the name doesn't say (probably because they ran out of space) is that it is also brightening and immediately lights up your face. And, when it is on, it has the resilience of Theresa May – completely unyielding – which is both good and bad. It is inflexible but for better or worse, will stay the course. The finish is also polarising and unapologetically matte (they call it demi matte, but it's matte). Choosing the shade is also tricky – do you know what Dark Neutral means? No, me neither – and the shade range is limited to fourteen, with the darker-shade offering not particularly extensive. So, not perfect, but if you are ever tempted to look up the definition of Full Coverage, don't bother. This is all the definition you need.

FENTY BEAUTY
Pro Filt'r Instant Retouch Concealer

Here we are congratulating brands with twelve, fifteen or twenty-max shades in their concealer line-up, and Fenty just comes in and shuts down the beauty industry by launching fifty shades: FIFTY. Five Zero. I mean, should I just stop writing now? Because that is EVERYTHING. You can tell I'm excited, right? I promise I am not doing that thing we all do when we type out a LOL/funny-face text-message response while looking completely deadpan. I am truly excited about it and not because I am sucked into the hype. I am excited because this is a fabulous product. I'll put my neck on the line and say that it is superior to even the foundation. Fifty shades of concealer is inclusive beauty on another level. Unless you are made up of floral-patterned stripes in acid hues, I can't see how you wouldn't find your shade here. The concealer itself is creamy and lightweight but gives you full coverage in a way that others don't. It covers dark circles, hyperpigmentation and blemishes well: a triple threat, if you will. It can be used in conjunction with a foundation or on its own. It can also double as a highlighter (a natural highlighter, not the sort that makes you look like a disco ball). You can use it as contour stick, too (hats off if you have the skills – and the time). And it lasts for ever (OK, not quite, but it will go the distance). The thing that most impressed me was just how illuminating this formulation is; you would think light-bulbs had been woven into its fabric. Can you see why I am excited about this one? Forget about your face coming alive: this is a resurrection.

YSL
Touche Éclat High Cover Radiant Concealer

I once worked for an editor who banned us from describing anything as iconic. I was baffled at first, but then I pondered it – as you do when someone says something that initially sounds wrong – and I understood. The word iconic has been overused, and now I am a little bit allergic to it. This concealer, however, does warrant the term. Touche Éclat is iconic. It's funny because, many moons ago, I remember hearing everyone (OK, not everyone, women. OK, not all women, Caucasian women) laud Touche Éclat – then, essentially, a highlighter – although a lot of people thought it was supposed to conceal, too. It didn't come in my shade, not even close, and the one I did try gave me reverse panda eyes. Every time anyone mentioned Touche Éclat I would feel like it was a conversation about the party of a lifetime to which I hadn't been invited. Fast forward almost two decades and the latest incarnation of the iconic (OK, I'll stop now, my former boss would be mortified) highlighter is a concealer, and it comes in an inclusive 16-strong range. Hurrah! We can all now join the party.

The USP is the anti-fatigue complex of caffeine and vitamin E and Ruscus extract. It covers dark spots, pigmentation and dark circles and, crucially, makes you look more awake (I find it particularly useful for the shadows around the mouth and nose). Then there are the light-generating pigments that, all of a sudden, lift your face so you become the embodiment of radiance. The texture is akin to a mid-weight creamy foundation. Don't be fooled by that, though. It dries quickly; after which it.does.not. budge. Which, of course, is a good and a bad thing: you have to be speedy in your application but, to be fair, it is quite hydrating so it won't be punishing on your creases. Now we need to talk about the utterly beautiful pen. When you become the proud owner of this, you will spot it in your bag and smile smugly as the voice in your head confirms how chic you are. It has a clicker at the bottom and a brush at the tip: you click and the product seeps out of the white brush. On first try, mind you, I had to click around 200 times before I saw an ooze of pigment. Never mind don't try this at home, don't try this in public: the noise will irritate the hell out of everyone.

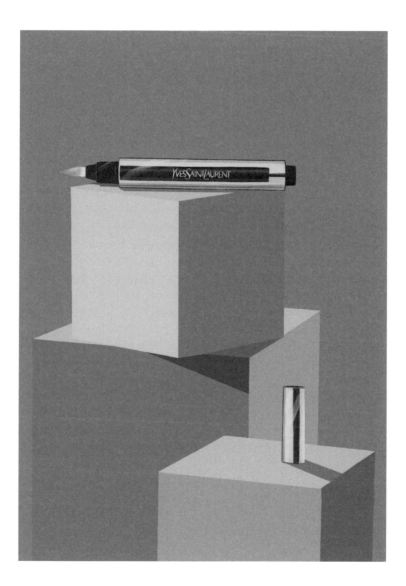

LAURA MERCIER
Flawless Fusion
Ultra-Longwear
Concealer

I first tried this at a time when everything that could go wrong did go wrong. I was internalising my stress – yes, the ultimate anti-self-care, but it was either that or go around screaming like a banshee. One day I looked in the mirror and wondered who was staring back at me. Like a good beauty editor, my first thought was, right, let's get some war paint on (because, of course, a made-up face is all you need to overcome the world's ills). That is how I discovered this concealer. I put it on, and, suddenly, I looked less decrepit. The hydrating formulation is clever, consistent and worthy of the name concealer, because it really does conceal (dark circles and pigmentation be gone!), and it does it for a while (for at least 12 hours), in the way that the best-dressed people say, 'What, this old thing?' It is all completely effortless. This is down to the technologically advanced formula, which is so ultra thin that it feels invisible on the skin, yet it does the job of a powerhouse.

It contains a Blurring Powder Blend that gives a soft focused finish of which Instagram would be proud. It also has a Skin-Fusion Technology that bonds polymers to the skin, so the concealer is resistant to sweat, humidity and water (which doesn't mean you can't wash it off; rather, if you got caught in the rain you wouldn't look like a drowned rat by the time you got to work). The shade range (twelve) is not huge, but it is well balanced between dark and light. The doe-foot applicator wand does feel flimsy on initial use, but after a while you realise that's no bad thing. It means the wand is more flexible, and the tip can get into those tricky crevices, like the edge of the nose, much more easily. What I love most about this concealer, however, is that it is oil-free. The last thing you need when you're having a terrible week is a greasy under eye.

COVER FX
High Performance
Setting Spray

A face mist and a setting spray are not the same thing. A mist should, at the very least, hydrate your skin. A setting spray on the other hand, sets your make-up so come 4pm you don't find yourself looking in the mirror horrified. It is important to make the distinction because many people buy mists in the hope that they double up as setting sprays. That's not to say a 2 in 1 is impossible but the majority do not have an effective dual function. You are better off with a straight-up face mist and a straight-up setting spray. If they come with added bonuses, even better. Hence I love Cover FX's setting spray. This sulphate-, paraben- and cruelty-free 'High Performance' product not only locks in your make up for up to 24 hours, it ticks other boxes without veering from its sole purpose. The nozzle is one of the keys to its success. It enables the product to be delivered in a fine mist. This is a dream; many setting sprays squirt a clumsy shower of liquid that ironically ends up destroying your make-up (#streakyface). The mist sets quickly without being drying and it is alcohol-free. Which is wonderful because no one wants a facial straitjacket. It's also non-sticky, the conditioning algae

protect skin from free radicals and airborne pollution and the oil-absorbing polymers make it a must for oily skins. Or for anyone that wants to go all day with their make-up totally intact – no fade down, no slipping, no cracks and no shift. You won't get this with a bog-standard mist. Therein lies the difference.

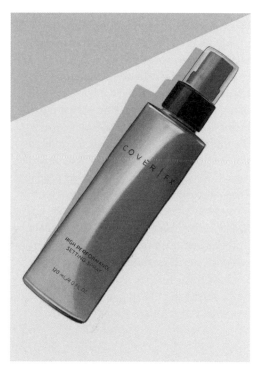

URBAN DECAY
All Nighter Long Lasting Makeup Setting Spray

In life, there are more pressing matters than whether your concealer has disintegrated into your creases. Even so, this is a first-world problem we could all do without. The last thing any of us want to do is keep rushing off to the ladies to fix a falling-apart face. To avoid that drama, I use this setting spray. I'm all about results and boy, does this deliver. If your make-up is war paint, then think of this 16-hour-hold setting spray as your added ammunition. I've used it on days that have kicked off with a crack-of-dawn breakfast meeting, followed by a flurry of appointments and ending with a fancy beauty industry dinner and party. Come the end of the night, I've been stunned to note my make-up has remained completely intact. This has a lot to do with its patented Temperature Control Technology, which lowers the temperature of your make-up to stop everything from melting off. The practicalities also make this spray superior to its peers – it comes in a nifty, travel-friendly mini version, the 'juice' comes out like a mist rather than a flood (so you're not left with water 'plops' all over your face)

and the tube is slimline, which makes it much easier to hold. Some may consider the alcohol in the formulation a downside, but it doesn't dry the skin out, so I would put that out of your mind. What's more important to remember is that this oil-free setting spray is so effective, your make-up could (almost) survive an apocalypse.

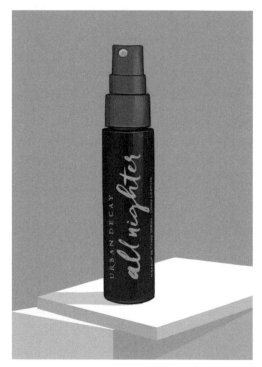

KAT VON D
Lock-It Setting Powder

I love a good setting powder but it is difficult to find one that doesn't take the joy out of your skin. I want a setting powder to give my make-up a polished finish and stop it melting into nothingness – one that kills the shine but not the glow. A powder should not leave a chalky film, it shouldn't be heavy, and it most definitely should not sink into your pores and creases. This powder meets every single criterion and more. It is so finely milled it feels like silk (it claims to be 45 per cent lighter than its best-selling competitor), it has a micro-blurring technology that perfects the look of your skin, it locks in your make-up and if you need to reapply – a rare occurrence – there is no caking. But do you know what's even better? It is translucent. As in properly translucent, so it actually works on darker skin tones, rather than claiming to be translucent while leaving you looking like you've dipped your face in cornflour. How much you love this powder may boil down to what sort of finish you want. If a full-on dewy look is your ride or die then you are better off sticking to a setting spray. If you like a bit of both, dab this only on the areas that typically get oily such as the forehead and nose. But if you have oily skin and heaven to you is a velvety matte finish, then prepare yourself for a love-in.

EYES

THINGS TO NOTE...

Once upon a time, you were advised to choose your eyeshadow according to your eye colour. Pah! Choose your shadows according to the strength of pigment and nail the application method; that will make all the difference. The same goes for brows, but, remember, jet-black brows are rarely ever a good look. Mascaras that simply give you a very natural look (read: as if you've got no mascara on) are not worth the money, and if you want a maximum-impact graphic eye, get an inky-black liner – anything less looks dead on our skin.

STILA
HUGE™ Extreme
Lash Mascara

I hate to be the bearer of bad news, but as you grow older, your lashes will go from being a fan made out of plush feathers to pitiful stumps of nothingness. What's scary is that you'll have no idea when it happens. Like death and taxes (unless you are Amazon or Starbucks) it eventually happens to us all. But if you don't want to spend your life buried under false lashes so huge you can't actually see where you are going, what's the alternative? Well, this. The clue is in the word HUGE™. And it delivers, although I do need to caveat this: the word huge is relative. As a child, my mother's shoes seemed huge. The point I'm making is, as always, rein in your expectations. How huge your lashes are with this depends on what state your original lashes are in. The key to judging the game-changing (or not) characteristics of a mascara is simply to try it on one eye first and then look at the difference. If it's barely visible, step away from the dud. With this mascara, however, you see an immediate lift with just one coat (and I managed to apply it without looking in the mirror – the ergonomics

of the wand is genius). The first thing you notice when you take out the wand is the sumptuous 'plop' sound it makes. This is always promising, because it hints at a rich, generous formulation. The shade is super jet black, like a Blackety Black Y'all black, which is wonderful because a semi/demi/off black just doesn't begin to touch the sides. The fat, curved brush comes out with quite a bit of product, thick and somewhat gunky, which does immediately make you think you will end up with clumpy lashes. Now, this sounds like an odd thing to say but I quite like the irreverence of clumpy lashes, although I know it's an acquired taste. But this won't clump your lashes at all – the blend of soft waxes builds the volume without the clump. The style of the brush mimics the eye shape and the wax formulation coats them accordingly and individually. Thanks to the lash conditioners, it doesn't crisp. This is always a good thing: no one wants a face covered in the remnants of crumbly mascara.

TOO FACED
Better Than Sex
Mascara

The suggestive name of this mascara came about because, apparently, it 'lasts all day long'. Sigh. I am a little bit over the retrograde cliché of sex sells. Also, can you recommend this without having some sort of conversation around it? Can I mention it to my older, beauty-obsessed aunt? With a straight face? OK, fair enough, a 79-year-old Nigerian grandmother is not their target audience, but you see my point. Ironically, the first time I used this, I went to bed wearing it. Me, the girl who desperately tries but fails to hide her horror if anyone admits to going to bed with slap on. What a hypocrite. But allow me to put some context to this. I wanted to try on this mascara, but I had already washed my face for the night. This means a number of steps had already taken place – cleanse, tone, liquid exfoliation, serum, vitamin C, glycolic, Q10, hyaluronic acid. I have my moments of being enthusiastic about my skincare, but even I wouldn't be able to muster the energy to carry out this ritual twice a night. But, call it a moment of abandonment, I put on the mascara, anyway – it was magnificent. I then faffed around, gorging on news and scrolling on Instagram, before I went to bed, knowing I'd either wake up sporting the insouciance of a supermodel post a night of partying (hopefully), or (more likely) looking twice as old. In reality, on awakening, the full luscious effects of the night before were slightly muted but still visible and, incredibly, my lashes were soft, and I had no smudges on my face or pillow. I put all that down to the groundbreaking formulation. This includes collagen to thicken, acacia senegal tree extract to boost volume, various peptides to condition and, polymers to lock curls into place, which is why you get those gloriously long, bushy and intensely dark lashes. The wand (perfect length, perfect width) makes it easy to apply across both eyes. The ingenious hourglass-shaped brush ensures just one coat spreads the satisfyingly sludgy texture evenly across the lashes, from root to tip. For more drama simply layer on more coats, which, because of the epic formulation, you can do without the fear of a flaky finish. This is everything you would want in a mascara. But, I hear you snigger, is it better than sex? Well, that depends on what sort of sex you're having.

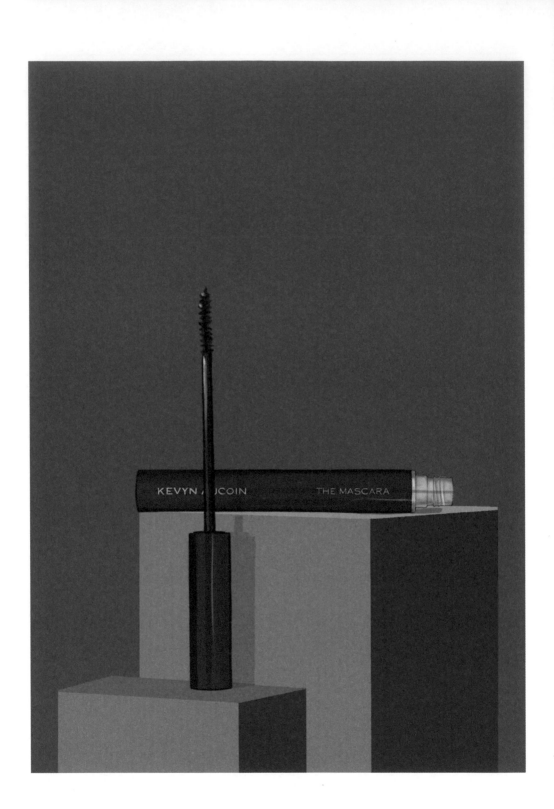

KEVYN AUCOIN
The Volume Mascara

The simple fact that this looks like a seriously upmarket pen brings me joy. But can I be honest? My heart sank when I opened it and saw it had a thin mascara wand. There is something about spindly wands that reminds me of having salad for supper – it leaves me wanting. I always feel that you have to be quite deft in your handling of a thin brush, which needs so much precision, whereas, with a big, fat brush, well, any old cack-handed person can handle that. If you can't cope with a spindly brush (it's very much a personal thing) feel free to move on, there's a world full of chubby brushes waiting for you. However, for those who have a predilection for skinny brushes, as you were.

This mascara has won serious plaudits from industry insiders, and there is a reason why. It works. You only have to look at your before and after to see what a difference it makes to your face. It thickens, it separates, lengthens and (jojoba oil) moisturises your lashes. If you are looking for a mascara that gives you that mega false-lash flutter, you are barking up the wrong tree. Yes, it is volumising, but in a natural way. There is no faux about it. It is not overly exaggerated, but you only have to use it on one eye to realise how pitiful your other eye looks in comparison. It says this is a 'one coat' mascara. I would say that if you want a more in-your-face effect, you will need more than that. While the lazy part of you might groan, the good thing with this is that it is completely buildable and adding more layers only increases the intensity and not the clogging potential. Another good thing, for all my moaning about a thin brush, this one allows you to get into the edges of your sparse lashes. An overweight brush won't do that; more accurately, it will do, but leaving smudges so you resemble an Eighties glam-rock star.

HOURGLASS
Caution™ Extreme Lash Mascara

I love this mascara. It is so major. Of course, the beautiful gold encasing is good eye candy but, essentially, the stuff inside it is brilliant. If you want no-holds-barred, high-impact lashes, come on in to the house of incredible length, volume and intensely inky lashes (this is not a mascara for wallflowers). The applicator is two brushes that have been moulded together in order to coat lashes from a 360-degree angle. The wand is a good length – not too long so you'd worry about poking your eyes out; nor too short so it becomes like trying to write a novel with a one-inch pen. So many mascaras have a 'one coat' claim; most do not deliver on that promise and should be done for false advertising. This, on the other hand, is the real deal. The clever formulation of hard and soft waxes means you achieve a bold finish super quickly.

It's buildable, too; and it doesn't budge or smudge. Actually, let me clarify that. Even the best mascaras will smudge if you do not apply them properly. What I mean is that once it's on, it's on. It has longevity so you won't look in the mirror halfway through the day and wonder why your mascara has scampered down your face.

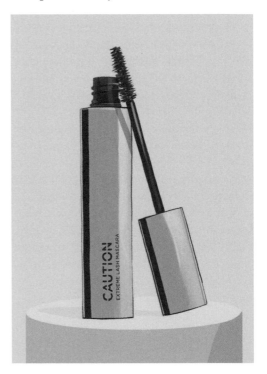

IT COSMETICS™
Superhero™ Mascara

In normal circumstances an extra-long mascara tube is a bit annoying. Unless your make-up bag is wide enough to accommodate a newborn, most of these mascaras would struggle to fit. I can forgive this mascara, however, because it is utterly superb. It is clinically proven to give you a flutter that is long, full, thick and beautifully black, that is, a black cape for your lashes. Surely this is what we all want? Have you ever heard anyone say, 'Oh, if only I had short, stocky, sparse lashes.' If you have lashes that seem hopeless, try this; even little stumpy hairs won't be able to resist the Elastic Stretch Technology. This stretches out your lashes so they look much longer and fuller instantly, which is great because, these days, mascaras that only do one or the other are not value for money. I don't want long lashes that have no volume, and I don't want full lashes stumpier than a bottle of stout. We're in the age of the hyphenate; we want it all, and this doesn't disappoint. It has been developed with plastic surgeons to include protein, peptides, biotin and polymers, all of which condition, strengthen and protect your lashes; hence it is known as 'skincare for your lashes'. But don't get too excited and expect it to smell like your favourite serum – it doesn't. It just smells like mascara; like really strong mascara, but it's not so odious to make you gag. The texture is gloopy, and I know a few people have complained that it can be messy. But, listen, if I, a beauty editor, whose idea of hell is getting her make-up incredibly precise, can apply this mascara and not end up looking worse for wear, so can you.

BENEFIT
They're Real! Lengthening Mascara / Benefit BADgal BANG! Volumising Mascara

There is something about gimmicky beauty products that seems supremely unsophisticated. The snooty part of you automatically begins making assumptions about the target audience (giggly, superficial and unsophisticated) and the quality (cheap, bad and unsophisticated). Then you feel so blissfully pleased with yourself because you think you've nailed it – until something comes along and completely throws out your preconceived ideas. Benefit has product names like Cheekleaders and Hello Flawless! It celebrated the launch of its winged eyeliner in a fried-chicken pop-up – it doesn't get more gimmicky than that. But to assume Benefit is fluffy, frivolous and inefficient would be daft. First, the brand does huge business, and, second, the technology that goes into its formulations and the results these produce are phenomenal. This is why any serious edit of great mascaras will always include BADgal BANG! and They're Real! (those are Benefit's exclamation marks, by the way).

Both these mascaras are serious players. Let's start with BGB (easier to abbreviate, no?). It's a 'BIGGER, BADDER volumising mascara'. I just love the way Benefit makes no bones about its merits. It's rather braggadocious but justified; the stats back it up: 90 per cent saw dramatic volume, 94 per cent said it instantly lifted lashes, and 93 per cent claimed it lengthened lashes. I can verify this, too: yes, I've seen all of that. It uses aero particles, developed from space technology, to add volume, length and curl to lashes. The wand is medium sized with a prickly, bendy rubber brush, which Benefit calls a Slimpact!; I think it looks like a skinny cactus. Anyway, there's obviously some sort of genius in the design, because it coats every single lash, from root to tip, from corner to corner, magnificently. You do end up with these dark luscious lashes you never knew could be yours (well, at least not without buying them anyway). It's also smudge proof, flake free and water resistant (you won't get caught in the rain and suddenly look like Alice Cooper's adopted sister).

If BGB! is Beyoncé's *Lemonade* then *They're Real!* is Solange's *A Seat at the Table*, the latter equally brilliant but less bombastic. They're Real! is perfect for those who cower at the thought of full-volume lashes. Like BGB, there are stats to back up its efficacy: it adds significant volume and definition to lashes and has a brilliant brush, so you can get into every nook and cranny to catch and lengthen even the most bitty lashes to the nth degree. Yes, we can call these mascaras gimmicky, but let's also call them brilliant because, bottom line, that's what they are.

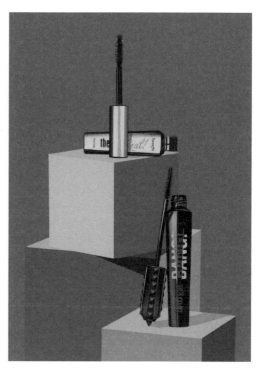

NARS
Climax Mascara

'**Reach your climax with explosive volume**': here, once again, is another **mascara with a sexually charged name.** At the risk of sounding pious, I am here sighing with my hand to my head. Perhaps it's because we have come to know NARS – a brand I love – as slightly edgy and subversive, that I've begun to expect it. After all, this is the brand that has normalised going to a make-up counter, poker-faced, and asking for an Orgasm (for those who don't know, it is their best-selling cult blusher/highlighter). I sigh because, naively, there's still a part of me that wonders, if you have a great product, is it necessary to use sex to sell it? Because this doesn't need that: it is a brilliant mascara. First of all, I love the ridged tubular packaging, not least because it looks both elegant and edgy but equally because it's bright red; you will always be able to spot it at the bottom of your bag. The wand is not too long, which makes it a cinch to use (anything too thin and too long, I find, requires a steady and expert hand that not everyone has). The full-bodied and bristly brush feels like it is combing your lashes with product. Created with a lash moisture complex, it is deeply pigmented (NARS calls it 'blackened') and goes on without creating clumps or smudges. When it dries, your lashes still feel really soft. Thankfully, every brand worth its salt is launching a formula with staying power without the stiffness; flaky lashes make you look like you haven't washed your face for a week. If you were looking for a lash lengthener, this wouldn't be my first port of call: volume is the USP here. But if you want soft, jet-black, full-impact lashes and are not jarred that the strapline is 'Hardcore Volume, Softcore Feel' then welcome this mascara to your world.

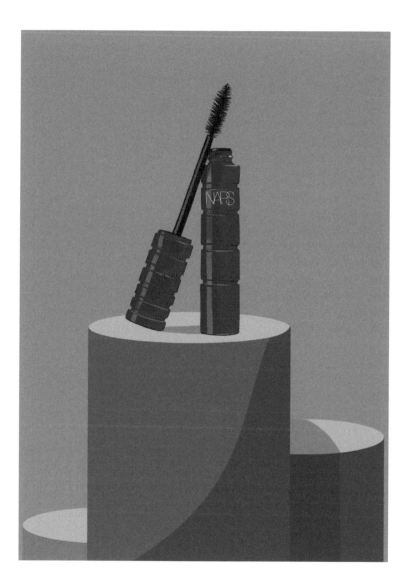

URBAN DECAY
Perversion Mascara

Is this name referencing S&M? I have racked my brain, and I honestly have no idea why this is called Perversion. My husband and I laughed at what we imagined would be the reaction if we showed this to one of my elderly African relatives. 'Ah, what is this?! Perversion?!!! God forbid! We rebuke it in Jesus name!!' The name may be polarising, but the quality and efficacy of the mascara is not in question. It is quite major. The packaging it comes in says Bigger Blacker Badder, and you know what? Tick, Tick, Tick. First, it is the type of brush to which I automatically gravitate, unapologetically big and fat. I'll admit, it does make it rather tricky to grab the little stray lashes without making a mess, so I would suggest having a stash of cotton buds dipped in make-up remover to hand, otherwise you will look like a raccoon. The formula is quite thick so avoid constantly pumping the brush into the tube or you will end up with too much product on the brush. While it says it is clump free, well, it's hard to avoid clumping due to the density of the formulation. However, it is nothing that can't be combed through – the brush is brilliant at separating and defining the lashes. The slower you are at applying, the less clumps you'll have to deal with. The final result is shiny – think latex – full-bodied lashes in an opaque blackness. Unless your idea of dress-down days always involves five-inch Loubies, this is not an everyday mascara and definitely not for the shy and retiring. A few things to note: for an even more dramatic finish, you can layer this formulation but, remember, it is not lightweight. If you go overboard, you might feel like you've got tarantulas for lashes. Although, thinking about it, for some people, that's a really good look.

CHANEL
Le Volume Révolution De Chanel Extreme Volume Mascara 3D-Printed Brush

Ah, Chanel. I rarely come across beauty products with as many names as your products. It's like looking at a Nigerian birth certificate. (For those who don't know, we have a million and one names.) Still, there are some names missing: 'impressive' 'innovative' 'incredible'... because this seriously is. Chanel is the first brand to market 3D mascara. The formula is a thick putty blend of rice wax, beeswax, vitamins and polymers but, in many ways, that's by the by, because they do say your mascara is only as good as the brush. And Chanel has aced it; the star is the brush. Patented more than ten years ago, it was made in collaboration with a best-in-class 3D-printing company, and the production processes are insane (they can print 50,000 brushes in 24 hours). The result is a brush with an incredibly precise original shape (to the naked eye, its trellis shapes probably look no different to any other but, trust me, this is next level). The 'granular texture' means your lashes adhere better to the product, and the formula is distributed on your lashes in a way that is more efficient, so there are no lumpy clumpy bits. There are microcavities on the brush, so it dispenses the right dose. You don't have to keep pumping the brush in and out of the tube to build lash volume (the less you dip your brush in and out, the less likely your mascara, indeed, any mascara, is to dry out).

OK, so that's the science bit over. What does it all mean in real talk? In a nutshell, you'll have transformed lashes in seconds. Seriously. You really don't have to work this one hard to get fuller, glossier, thicker lashes. The pigment is a wonderful inky black. The texture is quite thick, so there is a cynical side that wonders whether it will clump. But it doesn't. It does dry quickly but not crisply, so if you did decide to layer on some more, it won't flake or smudge. If you are seeking OTT look-at-me-spider lashes, this isn't that kind of party. It's more of a chic London cocktail do as opposed to grand debutante ball.

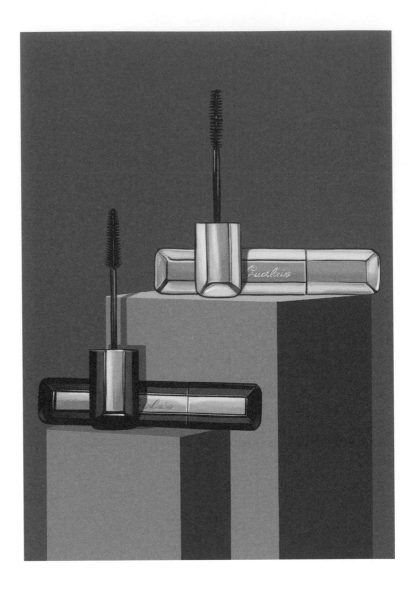

GUERLAIN
Cils d'enfer Maxi Lash So Volume Mascara / Volume Creating Curl Sculpting Mascara

It's funny what we accept and don't challenge despite not being particularly happy about it. This applies to big life issues as well as teeny, let's be honest, inconsequential stuff. For instance, I have tons of mascaras that I love, and because I love them so much I ignore the thing about them that niggles. My common-denominator bugbear is that archetypical mascara scent. Some are subtle, so just about bearable. Others, however, are so chemically pungent I find myself wrinkling my nose in irritation. Therefore, joy of joys, I was thrilled to discover these and find they don't actually smell like mascara *sings Etta James's 'At Last' really badly*. Instead, they are scented with jasmine, peach blossom and rose; they smell utterly divine. These have also won me over with their exquisite packaging – you will never again think mascara is a silly idea for a gift. The Curl one in particular is divine – it's like a bar of gold. Its compact size makes it an excellent travel companion, and the length of the brush is also a winner – so much easier to navigate around your eyes.

The difference between these two mascaras is not actually that significant but, put crudely, Cils d'Enfer So Volume lengthens and adds volume, but its real USP is the delivery of a great curl. If you're not brave enough to use an eyelash curler for fear of it clamping your eyes shut for ever (join the club), you'll love this. Lash So Volume is all about exactly that: volume. Someone described this as 'If Porsche made mascara.' Think expensive-looking glossy and 'look at me' lashes. Both mascaras have the benefit of a great, flexible brush with bristles that leave no lash behind and deliver an equal intensity of pigment. They both contain conditioning oils, which means you are less likely to get stiff crumbly lashes. However, I must caveat this. If you choose to layer and layer and layer, your lashes will flake. It is near impossible to overload them with this product without consequences.

BENEFIT
Goof Proof Brow Pencil/Gimme Brow⁺ Volumizing Eyebrow Gel

You'd think getting a brow pencil from the high street or a major brand – be it mass or prestige – would be pretty simple. I am stunned at the number of brow products I have received that are supposedly for 'you'. Unless for whatever reason I *wanted* to sport grey brows... because that is the only way I would be satisfied with most of the offering.. I'm sent browns that are never quite deep and warm enough. I'm sent an off black that gives me the aforementioned ashy brow. And then I get sent black. Sigh. I mean have you ever seen anyone who looks good with a jet-black drawn-in brow?! Anyway, one day a bag of Benefit brow products appeared on my desk, and I discovered the Goof Proof Brow Pencil. And angels started singing. It has a silky easy-to-use 'goof proof' tip (that never needs sharpening) in a glide-on formula. It makes getting precise brows really straightforward – honestly, any fool could use it. The best thing, of course, was the shade. It was spot on: a deep rich brown with no grey undertones. It's called Number 6. And that's the trick to getting your brow product right with Benefit – so long as you know your number, you just choose any of their brow products within their range, and it will be right. If you want fuller brows without that architecturally carved-out finish (that is, you have no desire for Instagram brows), Gimme Brow+ Volumizing Eyebrow Gel is a brilliant tinted gel that contains mini pigmented microfibres, which adhere to your brow hairs. The short brush needs no expertise, so in seconds you have tidy, glossier, thicker brows, which are natural looking and buildable. Not quite so buildable that it'll give you heavily pigmented 'angry brows', but if you are a fan of this product, I doubt you'd be that way inclined, anyway.

ANASTASIA BEVERLY HILLS
DIPBROW® Pomade/ DIPBROW® Gel

It might sound like an odd thing for a beauty editor to say, and I make no secret of this, but I find applying make-up laborious. Sorry, if I've disappointed you. Don't get me wrong, I love make-up (I'd be in the wrong job otherwise), and I don't feel like this every single day. But I do have days when the thought of applying a full maquillage makes me want to walk around with a T-shirt declaring, 'I really can't be arsed.' The element of my make-up that I find most tiresome is doing my brows. Getting brows right is an art. They say they shouldn't be twins (so they don't need to be identical), but they should be sisters. I have seen many women with brows that are enemies. Like I say, good brows take skill. But they also take good product. Anastasia's brow products make the process so much less stressful – and the results much more attractive. The Pomade is a thick, incredibly dense, well, pomade; a heavy texture that gives you seriously defined brows that are unbudgeable, come rain or shine. The pigment is rich,

and the texture is quite putty-like but, interestingly, it blends perfectly with your natural brows and matches your skin tone. (Obviously, you would have needed to choose the right one in the first place. I use Ebony, which gives a very dark, but not black brow.) There is, however, some level of skill necessary here. You do need a brow brush, a steady-ish hand and to be clear on the kind of shape you should have – take your foot off the pedal and you could easily end up with two horizontal apostrophes above your eyes. If you can master the application and you have good tools, this brow pomade is second to none. For those who want something easier and less dense, the DIPBROW® Gel is a dream. If the Pomade is the glammed-up older sister, consider this the breezy sibling. It still has the colour pay-off, but it tints the brow, adds volume and leaves you with a less dense finish. And it comes in eleven shades, which is currently the largest shade range in any brow gel. This is the fastest route to fabulous brows; no skill necessary.

SUMANBROWS
Microblading

I'm going slightly off piste here, because this is not a take-home product. But I didn't feel I could legitimately talk brows and not mention microblading, a treatment to give you the best brows ever. It essentially involves injecting pigment into the skin to create your perfect brow. I am often asked if it isn't simply a fancy new name for tattooing. No, it is not; microblading is a much more refined technique, in which fine needles are scraped across the brow to create hairlike strokes. Yes, needles are used but so is an anaesthetic to numb the area pre-treatment. What you end up with is something that is strikingly realistic, as opposed to looking as if a child has just gone rogue with a permanent marker. More and more places are springing up, claiming to offer microblading, but I wouldn't trust them too readily. The majority have no idea how to work with darker skin tones; if you leave your brows in the hands of just anyone, a marker-pen scenario, or worse, awaits.

Suman is the microblading specialist and my go-to. She is phenomenal and, as a woman of colour herself, understands how pigment works (and doesn't work) on darker skin tones. She also studies your face and brow shape to determine how best to create your new brows. What people want to know is whether microblading is painful. Well, it shouldn't be. As mentioned, your brows are numbed before treatment, and while the sound of the needle scraping against your brow is somewhat disconcerting, you shouldn't feel anything. If you can, Suman simply tops up the numbing agent. After the scraping, the pigment is added. Admittedly, this does sting somewhat, but it's low-level stuff and nothing that will have you screaming for deliverance.

The whole process takes a couple of hours and your new brows will last up to eighteen months. Just think, almost two years without faffing around with your brows! How quickly they fade depends on a number of things: if, like me, you regularly use acids in your skincare regime, that will have an impact; whatever the case, the fade is slow, subtle and absolutely normal. Oh, one more thing to keep in mind. Don't get upset when you look in the mirror post treatment and realise your brows look much darker. That is totally normal and not so bad as to terrify your colleagues. By week two, they will simmer right down.

L.A. GIRL
Inspiring Brow Kit

This is going to sound terrible, but it is rare for me to buy a beauty product from a mass brand. For the most part, it is down to a lack of trust about the efficacy of a lot of these mass-market products on darker skin tones. I remember the days of buying products in chemists and how shocked I was at how they translated on to my skin (badly). Now of course, you can get a plethora of brands in the black hair-and-beauty supply stores that cater to us, but, let's be honest, they vary greatly in quality. I discovered this kit in one of those shops (probably somewhere in southeast London) and bought it out of desperation. I just could not find brow products with the right amount of pigment and the right shade of pigment and finish (hence my section on brows is relatively small). My thinking was, 'This is less than a fiver; if it turns out to be rubbish, as long as it doesn't bring me out in the plague, it won't be the end of the world.'

Well, what a find. I loved it. The kit comes with two brown shades (there are three options of the kit, so choose whichever is more suitable), a highlighter, wax, a mini tweezers and a spoolie with brush for application. Quelle surprise, the latter two products are manageable but, of course, not top of the range – so invest in higher-quality versions. However, the powders are brilliantly pigmented and easy to apply, the tin is easy to carry around, and, if you are on a budget (or not), you can't turn your nose up at this.

WEST BARN CO.
Soapbrows®

This is such a strange product recommendation, although in a rather fascinating way. It is basically a technique whereby you use soap to give you fuller, more feathery-looking brows. And that's it. Sounds basic, right? Yet it has become a thing. Interestingly, it is a concept that goes back decades (it is also known as the Hollywood Brow). My first question with so many of these types of trends is: 'Does it work on people of colour?' Unequivocally, yes; once you start using it, you'll become obsessed. I certainly have. It really is incredible. You can use any soap (clear not opaque), but seeing as this astute brand has packaged up an old-school technique in a portable tin, I thought it was worth a mention. The soap is a clear gold and smells like the original African black soap (Ose Dudu) with which my grandmother used to bathe us. The way it works is this. Take a glass of water, a spoolie (the eyebrow-brush thing; try to buy one that is not too big), dip it in some water, scrape it across the soap and begin to use it to brush up your brows. Your brows immediately look feathered, thicker and lush. You can fill in any gaps with your favourite brow products.

If you don't like a full fluffy-brow look and prefer something with a bit more definition, define under the brow with a brow product. Avoid drawing a line across the top – it will end up looking blocky and unnatural. Unless you've mastered the art of this technique, it is worth applying your foundation afterwards so you don't end up with a face with a soapy base. The amount of soap you need depends on your brows – the curlier they are, the more you will need – but start small and see how you fare. Nevertheless, try not to go too overboard and use masses of soap. If you do, it'll dry and you'll look as if you have a serious dandruff problem.

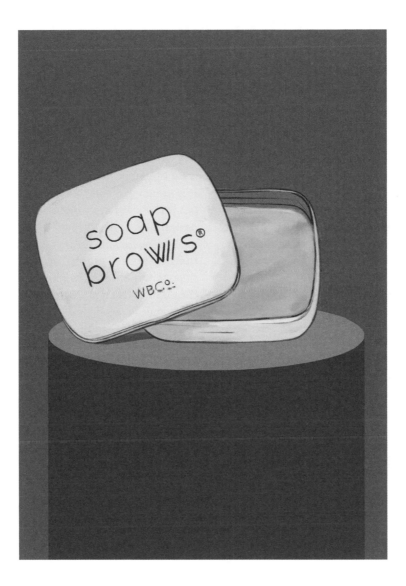

SMASHBOX
Brow Tech
Shaping Powder

Now, if you are the sort of person who wants a brow product that doesn't require any kind of precision, stop reading. It's not that this product is difficult per se, but it does take getting used to. It also requires a lot of patience, which, in the mornings, I don't have in spades, particularly if I'm just starting my make-up, the news beeps go off on Radio 4, and I realise I should have been on the train 15 minutes ago. This is literally a brow powder in a tube with a super thin applicator. If you struggle with the intricacies of liquid eyeliner, you might just hate this product. If you are a liquid-liner queen, well, this is a dream. A fine loose-pigmented powder (watch for spillages), it creates fuller, bolder brows in a natural way. It comes with a skinny liner applicator that you dip into the powder and paint onto your brows to boost their volume and fill in any patches or gaps. You see why you need a really steady hand? It is amazing for the feathered-brow look, but if you want more definition around the peripheries of your brows, use an eyebrow pencil as a finishing touch. I had concerns that this powder would have a tired grey tinge to it, but I was happily surprised – the pigment is on point and the texture silky smooth. If you are one of those people who can't even draw a straight line with a ruler, I wouldn't bother; this does not have your name on it. Ideally, it would be great if the shade range were extended, the liner weren't so intimidating, and speckles of powder didn't sometimes fall around your brow. But if you can deal with the application process, it is a keeper.

FENTY BEAUTY
Moroccan Spice
Eyeshadow Palette

Despite the huge noise and high-profile launches around Rihanna's beauty brand, it took a while before I got the chance to sit and have a play with the Fenty Beauty collection. I missed the original launch breakfast. I cannot remember exactly why, but I would wager it had something to do with a deadline. Shortly after that, the Chief Operating Officer of Harvey Nichols invited me to come and immerse myself in the brand. I took in the mammoth line of young girls who had been waiting for hours to get to the Fenty counter, and I didn't want to use my press privilege to jump to the front of the queue. When the actual launch party happened (you know, the one that Rihanna attended, wearing that cute Molly Goddard dress), it was like trying to swatch make-up in a nightclub: loud, dark, and impossible.

Finally, one early morning in front of London's King's Cross St Pancras station, Rihanna's team – including her brilliant make-up artist Priscilla Ono – set up a pop-up shop. I headed there, and, at last, I was able to try everything, in the light and at my leisure. The one thing that stood out that day was the Moroccan Spice Eyeshadow Palette. This 16-colour strong palette is stunning. The textures are mind-blowing: silky smooth with rich pigments, which are incredibly long wearing. Even by the very end of the day, the pigment hadn't dissipated; it is like ink. The colour mix is really wearable. There are browns, bronzes and golds as well as other pops of colour, such as dark greens, reds and peaches, in matte, shimmer and metallic finishes. They are all suitable across all skin tones. If there is a downside, then teeny first-world problem, it's the size, which is massive. But then that's Rihanna, isn't it? She doesn't do anything small.

URBAN DECAY
Naked Reloaded
Eyeshadow Palette

On the one hand, make-up palettes make complete sense. They are an excellent opportunity to experiment with lots of different colours, often at an accessible price point. On the other hand, most eyeshadow palettes comprise a few colours you would wear on a regular basis, some you might wear for a special occasion and, then, a handful you would never dream of wearing unless your life was at stake. Urban Decay's Naked Reloaded palette, however, is one of the first to be filled with colours that people want to wear. When the brand launched the original Naked palette, it was, let's just be straight here, for Caucasian skin. I am not for one second saying that this was on purpose; what I am saying is simply fact. And, to be fair, while not correct, that was the norm at that time: not many brands were thinking particularly inclusively. The colours were 'nudes', a word that has long been anathema to me, because there was never a nude that I recognised as mine.

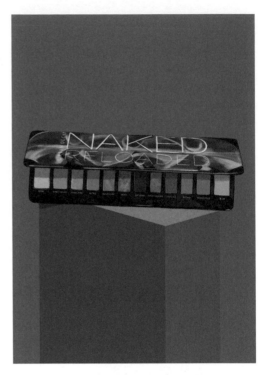

However, the Naked Reloaded eyeshadow palette has been completely revaluated and relaunched to incorporate twelve shades that speak to every skin tone. Universally flattering, these little rectangular pockets of joy come in browns, peaches, chocolate, rose golds; basically, in all the shades that more or less suit everyone. The texture is divine: the velvety mattes, iridescent shimmers and micro-shimmers all glide across your skin. The pigment is discernible and stays put all day. If you are going to invest in an eyeshadow palette, I can't think of one that offers better value for money.

CHARLOTTE TILBURY
Eyes to Mesmerise Cream Eyeshadow

There are tons of make-up artists with their own make-up line, but experience tells me that some of the most lauded make-up artists still have no idea what to do with darker skin tones. And so they create make-up lines that consider darker skins as an afterthought, if at all. Lipsticks are not too problematic (the 'nude' issue is ongoing), but everything else is a nightmare. The textures are all wrong, the pigments non-existent and good luck with trying to find your foundation shade. Charlotte Tilbury, however, is on a different level. She is one of the biggest make-up artists in the world, used to working on numerous skin tones; so her products generally work on darker skins. They also look good. I am all about beauty products that are, yes, beautiful, exciting and different, but, for me, ease is the greatest thing. Why would you want to make your life harder? Hence I recommend Eyes to Mesmerise, which are incredible mini pots of perfection. The formula is a whipped-up, water-infused cream that is highly pigmented, great for hydration and infused with vitamin E. It won't drag on your skin, and it is foolproof. For a wash of colour, use your fingertips to blend over your eyelids. For a more intense finish, use a brush. Choose from eight pots, of which my personal faves are Star Gold and Mona Lisa. They melt onto your skin like butter and feel as if they were made with your skin in mind, which I believe, beauty founders, is not too much to ask.

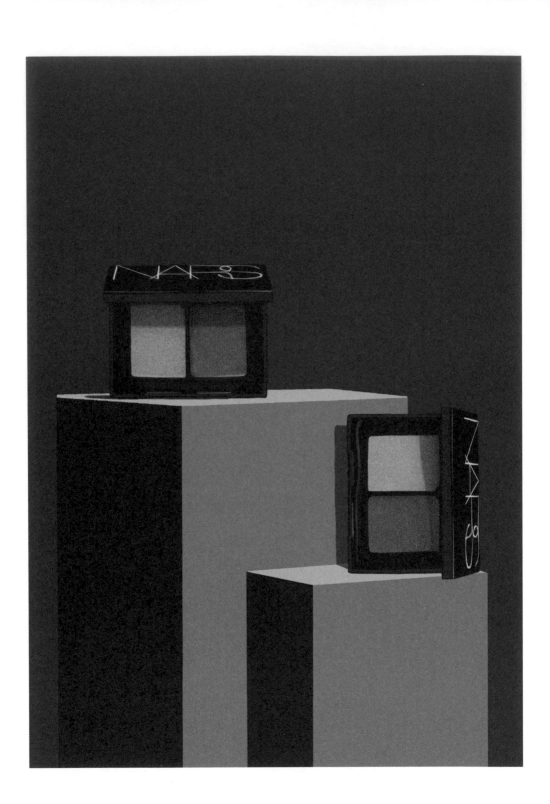

NARS
Duo Eyeshadow/ Eye Paint

This is dedicated to all those a little bit scared of eyeshadow. I see you watching, vicariously, from the sidelines. I myself am not a huge eyeshadow fan. Actually, that's not entirely true; so let me rephrase it: I am not a huge eyeshadow wearer, for many reasons. I have had too many experiences of someone convincing me that a shadowed eye is the way forward (more fool me); then just ending up resembling a black Grayson Perry. I've also seen how the overzealous application of eyeshadow can distort a person's face. And it is alarming. I remember meeting up with a friend who, after following the tips of a YouTube video, had blended a cacophony of hues over her eyelids. Honestly, she looked like an extra from *The Lion King* musical.

Another, quite key, reason I hold back on eyeshadow is fundamentally because I have never learnt to apply it with any level of proficiency. If it is a case of just swiping something across my lower lid, then that's fine. If I have to start blending and mixing, forget about it. Yet, when I look at the eye colours NARS has to offer – wonderfully pigmented colours, textures and finishes (matte, shimmer, metallic), crease-resistant and long-wearing – I long to master the art. In the meantime, I've discovered you can utilise eyeshadow in a way that does not involve intricate blending. These NARS shadows are versatile formulas that can be used wet or dry. A less intimidating approach is to take a damp brush (damp not soaked), stroke it across the eyeshadow of your choice and brush it across the top of your lid to give you a simple but modern pop of colour. As your confidence builds, you can experiment a bit more. Some of the duo eyeshadows worth trying include Surabaya (an incredible shimmering Brown Sugar and Chestnut), Kauai (Gold Foil and Iridescent Orchid), and Kuala Lumpur (Rose Gold and Boysenberry infused with Gold).

If you are looking for full-on pigment, the Eye Paints are incredible. These are super silky pots of pigment in an 18-hour long-wear gel format. They come in matte and metallic finishes (Ubangi, a black with blue shimmer, is insane), and they can be worn as a liner or a shadow. They are also beautiful on the skin (cheers, pomegranate and vitamin E), but, as before, unless you are auditioning for *The Lion King*, try not to use them all at once.

KEVYN AUCOIN
The Exotique Diamond Eye Gloss

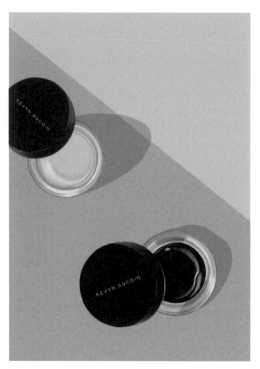

I've always admired the traditional smoky eye you get using eyeshadows. There is something about a dark smoky eye that is so undeniably covetable. It is sensual, sexy, and super cool. Well in theory anyway. On me, the whole thing is lost in translation. Creating the perfect smoky eye is all to do with astute blending and, just like baking, it is a skill that completely evades me. Doesn't matter how many 'How to Get a Smoky Eye' features I try to replicate, it takes me more time than I can afford to spare and I still end up looking like an ageing drag queen. Annoyingly, people assume beauty editors also moonlight as make up artists. That's like expecting war reporters to become soldiers. Anyway, I stopped trying to nail the perfect dark eye and I simply continued to admire people that are not as cackhanded with eyeshadows. And then I stumbled upon this black gloss with shimmering gold bits. It is in this pot of genius that I discovered a surprisingly wearable modern take on the smoky eye. And yes, this is a gloss that has been specifically created for the delicate eye area so it is quite literally easy on the eye. For everyone or anyone who has never been able to get on with the intricacies of eyeshadows, (surely it's not just me?) this pot of gloss is a godsend. It is embarrassingly easy to apply – I literally use my finger to slather it across my inner lid and then I dip a thin brush in the pot and apply around my lower lash line. Voila. Smoky eyes in 5 seconds flat. Two things to note. 1. While tempting, don't try lip gloss as an eye gloss, you need something created specially for the eye area, otherwise pain and irritation await. 2. I heard a rumour this this may be discontinued at some point so just in case; stockpile.

CHANEL
Stylo Ombre Et Contour Eyeshadow/Liner/Kohl

Does anyone remember Rouge Noir nail varnish? It is the deeply dark burgundy-ish, purple-ish, blood-red almost black shade that came to define the 1990s. It made its debut at Paris Fashion Week and, as a nail colour, epitomised the ultimate in everything cool, chic and sophisticated. Of course, it became highly coveted (even Uma Thurman wore it in *Pulp Fiction*, which, for the benefit of those who think, So?!, was quite major back then). It kept selling out, and you'd have to be put on a waiting list. Finally, I got my hands on one. This was the first item I ever bought from Chanel, and I was beside myself with joy. I've never loved a nail varnish more – I kept it in the fridge, for goodness' sake. And I wore it with immense pride, walking around flashing my hands about, smug and self-satisfied at being able to get hold of one in the first place. Those were the days when people went out and bought nail polish – I can't remember the last time I did that. Still, even all these years later, it is difficult for me to come across Rouge Noir and not feel a wonderful sense of nostalgia.

Hence I got incredibly excited about this multi-tasking 3-in-1 pen, which comes in the exact colour of my old-school nails. For someone who, generally, considers a palette of eyeshadows as an *objet d'art* (yes, it's pretty, but what on earth am I supposed to do with it?), anything that gives me a hint of colour without effort has my name all over it. This stick is creamy and silky, and glides over skin to leave a beautifully rich burgundy pigment that stays that way all day long. You can use it as an eyeliner (the pointy tip enables you to create shapes with precision), you can use it as an eyeshadow, and you can use it as a smudgy kohl. The wonderful thing about this colour is that it gives you a sexy, smouldering eye that doesn't look too much but ups the ante from the requisite black, which, to be fair, can sometimes be a little hard. That's my thinking, anyway. The stick's not particularly huge; if you use it every day don't be surprised if you suddenly realise it has turned into a stump. So, no, it doesn't last as long as a Duracell battery, but it is fabulous, and so it's worth it. I dare you not to want it in every colour.

PAT MCGRATH LABS
Bronze Seduction Palette

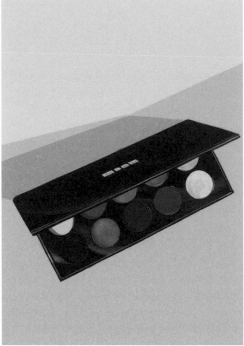

I have a difficult relationship with eyeshadows. I admire a good eye game on other women, but I personally don't have the patience to perfect the application process. However, even I find these irresistible. This heavyweight palette – literally, it weighs a ton – was created by an industry heavyweight, Pat McGrath, who is easily the biggest and most influential make-up artist in the world. With her work on the catwalks and on social media, Pat is one of the very few make-up artists who can legitimately call herself a trend-setter. I say this in part to help understand why you will find this more expensive than your run-of-the-mill palettes: this is the Aston Martin of its genre. Most palettes include a few duff colours most people will never wear, but the shades included in this one – browns, bronzes, deep aubergine – suit everyone and are incredibly easy to wear, even if you normally find eyeshadows scary. It does also include some more experimental colours, such as the intense bronze-toned orange, but they are still workable. The biggest draw, however, is the quality of the formulations. Pat herself swatched these colours on my skin and the density of them blew my mind. They glide on with ease and you only need a small amount, so the Second Coming may descend before you hit pan. Although be aware that the intensity of the pigment means it DOES NOT BUDGE. It lasts all day (and all night) so you will need to go to town to make sure it comes off. But do you know what? I don't think that's such a terrible problem to have.

LAURA MERCIER
Caviar Stick Eye Colour

I have never made any secret of the fact that I find 'doing my brows' a pain. The patience and precision it takes to get that perfectly sculpted brow on a daily basis just flummoxes me. And then there has been a deluge of trial and error with numerous brow products that are the wrong texture, wrong finish and, surprise, surprise, the wrong colour. When one day I desperately needed something to fill in the gaps this was to hand. Now, if you are going to use it on your brows, there are a few things you should know. It is not a brow pencil; it does not have the texture or finish of a brow pencil. If you use it on your brows, and you forget and rub your face, you will look in the mirror at the end of the day and realise you have been walking around with weird dark smudges on your face. You will find you have one eyebrow noticeably more balding and thinner than the other. So long story short, my experiment failed badly. The colour is beautiful, but it is incredibly dense. Unless you use a brow brush and cover the sparseness of your brows with painstaking attention to detail, you will just look like you have two strips of duct tape across your brows.

So I would suggest sticking to what this was created for, because, in that context, it is awesome. If you want a smoky, mussy rock-and-roll eye, this is how you get it. I love that kind of eye, but the products that achieve it in a way that translates onto darker skins are few and far between. The intensity of the Smoke pigment is divine. I also love Peacock, Plum and Sapphire. The texture is soft and slightly mushy, so it is best for that sexy 'morning after the night before' look (if you are looking for a defined winged eye then this won't work). It is smudgy, which is good and bad. You'll need a light touch in order to minimise the clean-up process (keep cotton buds to hand); it is a teeny bit fragile, so if you press too hard, it will eventually break off. It says it is non-transferable, which I don't really understand, given that the only eye make-up that lends itself to that is a decent liquid liner. This doesn't dry like ink. If you rub your eyes, don't expect it to stay put. That said, once it is on, so long as you don't tamper with it, it will stay on. Just don't be tempted to use it on your brows.

URBAN DECAY
24/7 Glide On Eyeliner

Magic. That's what these pencils are. They are the reason I first fell for coloured eyeliners. Vice (a shimmery aubergine), Sabbath (a matte deep navy) and Overdrive (a deep metallic green) are my favourites but there are 35 colours so explore away. Like with coloured mascara, many still find coloured eyeliner retrograde or simply unwearable, but I disagree. Worn the right way (i.e. by dialling down other aspects of your make-up) coloured eyeliner looks thoroughly modern and is an easy way to wear an eye colour without the all-or-nothing commitment and technique necessary with eye shadows. The pigment in this product is superb – creamy, waterproof, long-lasting and gloriously intense, which is necessary for creating an impact on darker skin tones. The semi-solid, gel-like texture is soft and pliable and glides on, as the name suggests, like silk,

giving you a really lovely, subtly smudgy finish. The nib is relatively small so if you want a quick-to-deliver punchy smudge, a big kajal pencil would be more appropriate. But if you want a softer line, you're in perfect company. Despite my adoration for these pencils, I do however have a couple of gripes. The pointy nib seems to go flat very quickly so you do have to consistently sharpen. My second complaint is that it doesn't come with a sharpener. Many do these days and I wish all brands would follow suit. Still, considering how often you need to sharpen these, they last an incredibly long time. See, I'm telling you. Magic.

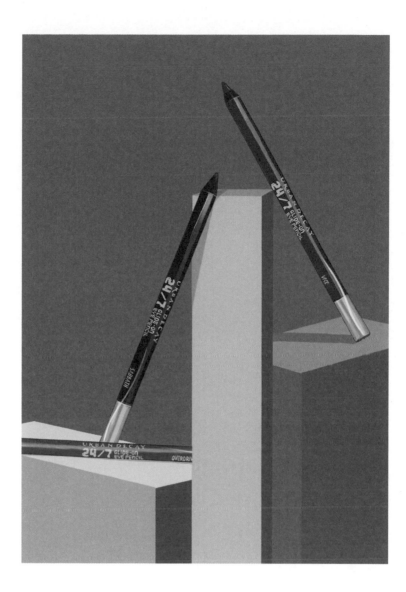

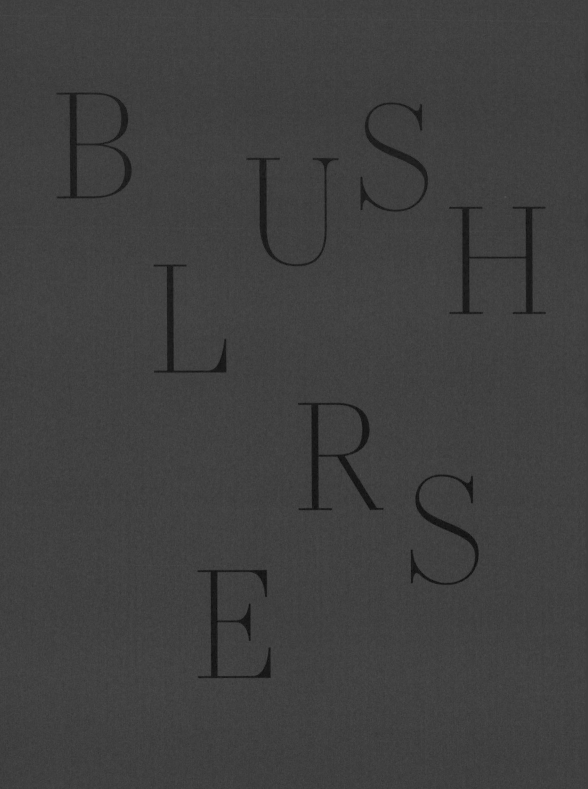

BLUSHERS
BUSH
BLUR
E

THINGS TO NOTE...

A cream blusher on top of a creamy
foundation? Good luck with that.
Whatever anyone tells you, it never
works. Neither do wishy-washy colours,
nor anything without a deep, rich
pigment. A powder blusher is perfect
for all skin tones, but dry skins must be
kept hydrated to stop any powder from
falling through the cracks.

MAC
Powder Blush

There was a time in my life when I had a thing for blushers. I would search high and low for the right one. It had to be pink but the right sort of pink. I would scrutinise photographs of celebrities wearing pink blushers and think, Yes! That's exactly the kind of blush situation I'm going for. Alas, it's difficult for sales people on make-up counters to translate that to black skin when you are holding up a still of Britney Spears from *Oops! ... I Did It Again*. Finally, though, I discovered my perfect pink powder blusher at MAC (it's been discontinued but it was akin to a deeper Pink Swoon). And I am sure anyone can find their blush here, because the shade range is ridiculously extensive. If you struggle to find any blusher you like then you are either not really a blusher person or the most difficult person on earth, and God help your loved ones. These epitomise the perfect matte blush. They are powdery (but not ashy), pigmented (but not overly intense) and silky smooth (so they sit beautifully on your skin and not in your pores). The MAC range has easy-to-wear shades as well as those that encourage you to leave your comfort zone. Raizin, a now cult golden reddish-brown, is the shade that make-up artists reach for when working on darker skin tones. It is also the shade I spot on huge numbers of women of colour. While Raizin complements our skin tone beautifully, I find it a little predictable, stereotypical and, dare I say it, unimaginative to automatically make a beeline for this. I can imagine the voice in the artist's head, 'She's black, she wants a blusher, I know, I'll give her Raizin.' So then everyone is walking around with the same cheek colour. This is why, unless I am asking for foundations or concealers, I no longer invite beauty companies to send a selection suitable for darker skin tones. Invariably, what they send boils down to brown lipsticks and brown blushers, shades I would never wear.

So, I encourage you to step out of the box and try other shades of blushers here. The formulations are exquisite; there is no need to fear that brighter shades will get lost in translation. Fashion Frenzy (a bright pink), for instance, looks scarier in the pot than it is. It immediately lifts the skin, makes you appear more youthful and looks great in hotter climes. Apple Red (a beautiful bluey red) is one that you might need to go light on as it is very red; it is, however, perfect for deep skin tones. If you prefer something a little more toned down, try Burnt Pepper, a dirty tangerine, or Diva Don't Care. It's a deep, rich burgundy that is a halfway house between something that totally blends in with your skin (yet, what's the point of a blush you can't really see?) and something that gives you that pop of colour. I don't care for the name or its connotations, but if you are looking for a blush that is simultaneously glamorous and understated, this is spot on.

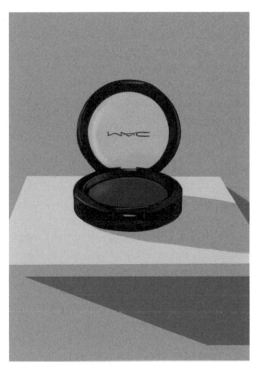

LAURA MERCIER
Blush Colour Infusion

It is interesting, the number of blushers that look like a good shot of colour, and yet when you try them, they disappear into your skin or leave an ashy finish. Laura Mercier's Blush Colour Infusion is one of the few that, on first impression, I thought might be a let-down. On closer inspection, however, it comes up trumps (yes, I'm aware that the use of this word has irrevocably changed). It is a 10-strong range of micro-fine solid powder blushers that leave skin silky smooth. The range of colours goes from Ginger, a matte 'nude', to Kir Royale, a matte berry red. What's clever about this range is that all the shades, bar none, have been created to work across all skin tones. Now they are not intensely heavy pigments but purposely created to have a sheer finish. The end result, therefore, is delicate, making them perfect for everyday wear or for when you need to inject a natural but long-wearing hint of colour. They are buildable; it's important, however, to be realistic: you can layer on as much as you like, but it would be unfair to expect them to deliver the kind of punchy pigment some brands do as a basic. Laura Mercier is not the kind of brand that shouts; more of a confident whisper, exactly what this blush is.

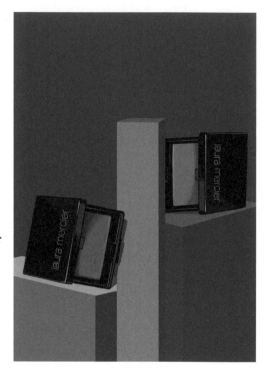

BOBBI BROWN
Blush

I've had many frustrating experiences of unsuccessfully trying to open a blusher compact, so it is an utter joy to be faced with the ease of this blusher. That is the wonder of Bobbi Brown: elegant and uncomplicated. People think of it as the brand you go to for everyday make-up. And, yes, it is, but limiting what it does to 'everyday' make-up, which sounds so dull, does it a disservice. It is so much more than that. The quality, range and finish could easily go toe to toe with brands that are much more vocal about their merits. So if you are looking for a true matte blush and want something straightforward and natural (not a purple blusher, though why would you want that anyway?) with a confident colour pay-off, you'll find it here.

Most of the fourteen-strong range would suit darker skin tones. My favourites are New Poppy (a red berry), Rose (a dark rosy red), Tawny (a pinky brown) and Apricot (more an orangey red than traditional apricot). It provides a fresh watercolour finish, which is the genius thing about this powder: it blends so beautifully that it is almost impossible to overdo it. OK, actually, maybe it isn't, but you'd have to go out of your way to get it really wrong. For those who have never used a blusher or feel nervous about it, this is a gentle but solid way to dip your toe in. Plus you won't have to spend fifteen minutes trying to work out how to open it.

SLEEK
Make Up Blush
By 3 Palette

Blushers are essentially crushed powders which could easily come in any colour, so you would think that, unlike a high-tech skincare product, it shouldn't take decades of research to deliver a decent one. And yet evidence points to the contrary. The prevailing issue amongst blushers is a lack of strong pigments and quality: a good blusher shouldn't accentuate inconsistencies in the skin. It shouldn't sit in your pores. And God forbid it should separate. I've seen a few bad blushers in my time and because the majority have been mass market, I had more or less written off inexpensive brands. Shame on me because these palettes are excellent, combining three complementary, highly pigmented shades – two matte, one shimmer – and a mirror to boot. With their incredible depth of pigment and a silk-like texture, the quality is equally as impressive.

Flame, a trio of toffee, deep orange (similar to NARS, Exhibit A) and shimmery brown red, is divine on darker skins, as is Sugar which comes with a stunning matte plum, shimmery golden brown and matte pale peach. I feel the latter is unsuited to darker skin but I'd suggest buying it just for the darker hues. Lace, a trio of peachy shades, works on lighter skins as does the cream blush variant Californ.I.A, although if you use this, skip your foundation to stop it turning to mush. Also beware that the pigments are high impact, so be sparing to avoid clown territory: it is easier to dial up than to dial down, so a layering approach is best for a more natural finish. Finally, don't suddenly assume all inexpensive blushers are superb – they are not. Sleek is in a category of its own.

NARS
Blush

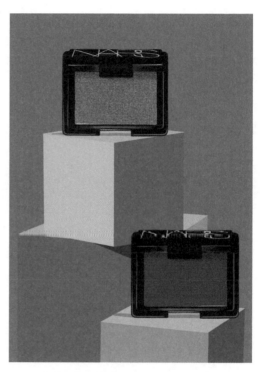

NARS calls itself 'The Ultimate Authority in Blush', and, you know, I totally get it. NARS has a right to say that because there is no blusher colour, finish or texture that you can't find under its wing. Orgasm is the one that has amassed a global cult following. This is probably its most famous product and the one where grown-ups still can't help looking embarrassed when they say the word. It is a pinky-gold shimmery powder with a silky finish that also comes in a liquid blush. Now, I struggle with liquid and cream blushes. Don't get me wrong: these are some of the best you can buy, and, on lighter skins, yes, they work well, leaving a beautifully dewy, pinkish shimmer. On darker skins, however, you would struggle to get a true representation of colour. Taj Mahal (a shimmering burnt-orange sibling, in a powder) would probably fare better, especially, if you were going to wear a foundation.

I would always recommend a powder blush over a cream or liquid one because, regardless of which colour you use, your blusher will end up brown. If you are darker skinned and looking for a straightforward pink blush with no shimmer, bypass Orgasm. The gold flecks of shimmer can overwhelm the pink; I feel it is more effective as a highlighter. A good matte option is Desire or Mata Hari, both beautiful pinks with incredible colour pay-off. If you prefer a deeper shade, Seduction is an exquisite burgundy matte with a soft sheen. There's also Exhibit A, a deeply intense orange that lifts even the dullest of demeanours. You will only need a light sweep of this colour. So you don't have to be heavy handed, otherwise you'll be mistaken for an ambulance siren.

LIPS

THINGS TO NOTE...

The way the beauty industry's going,
old-fashioned creamy lipstick bullets
will become extinct. OK, maybe not.
But go to any department store and you
will be bombarded by a mob of liquid
lipsticks in matte. Always look out for
hydrators in the formula and base your
lips with a lip primer, because while
most lipsticks won't dry your lips to
a crisp, some will.

BEAUTY PIE™
Fantasticolour Liquid Lipstick

Lately I have observed that the ratio of liquid lipsticks that land on my desk compared to the old-school lipsticks I receive is roughly around 10:1. 99 per cent of the lip colours I use are liquid lipsticks. I love the (predominantly) matte finishes, the ease of use, how you don't need to open them to get a sense of the colour, and how they don't melt in the heat. Of course, not all liquid lipsticks are equal. Some are so thick and unyielding they drag across your lips; others are so flimsy you would struggle to get a consistent colour pay-off, and many leave you with a cracked dryness that feels like a sprinkling of lead shavings. Beauty Pie joins a coterie of brands I feel have perfected the liquid lipstick. There are only six shades at present (essentially pinks, nudes and burgundy), which I find too narrow. However, that aside, it is impressive on many levels. The texture is a velvety matte (as opposed to a drying matte) that glides on effortlessly. It feels so light and conditioning – it is chock-full of coconut oil – and the pigment packs a punch. If you prefer a more toned-down finish, just applying less, with the simple but effective curved applicator, will deliver the results you require. Membership is worth investing in to gain access to the best luxury-beauty products, made in the world's best labs for up to five times less than standard prices, minus retailer mark-ups. You don't need a maths degree. It's a no-brainer.

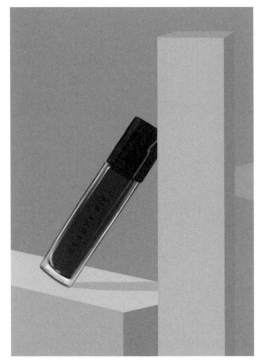

KAT VON D
Everlasting Liquid Lipstick

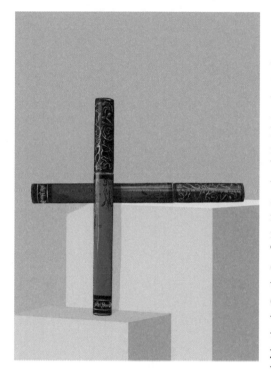

When you think about a cruelty-free, vegan, 'natural' make-up brand, how do you envisage it? Well, I'll tell you what I tend to see: airy-fairy, wishy-washy, barely there stuff that fails to pack a punch. But, of course, that's all OK, because it's saving the world. The thing that gets me is that so many small brands have a strange idea that just because they are 'natural', they have to be insipid. This is why I have to hand it to Kat Von D. She is so completely left of centre and proves the importance of thinking out of the box and doing something unexpected, hence her strong brand. The packaging might not be everyone's cup of tea: Goth-inspired beauty is not *my* spiritual home. However, this liquid lipstick was one of the first and is still one of the best. It's velvety and includes vitamin E and sunflower seed to make it glide effortlessly across your lips. There are colours from the usual suspects (pinks, reds, nudes) as well as the more technicolored and wonderfully bizarre (from bright purple to olive green). The wand is long and thin, so if you are used to working with a shorter applicator then you'll have to pay attention to avoid giving yourself a colourful moustache. On the strength of the colours alone, it is worth the risk. The fifty-plus shades are perfect for darker skin tones – so much so that even after you have taken it off, the stain is still very much visible. Everlasting for real.

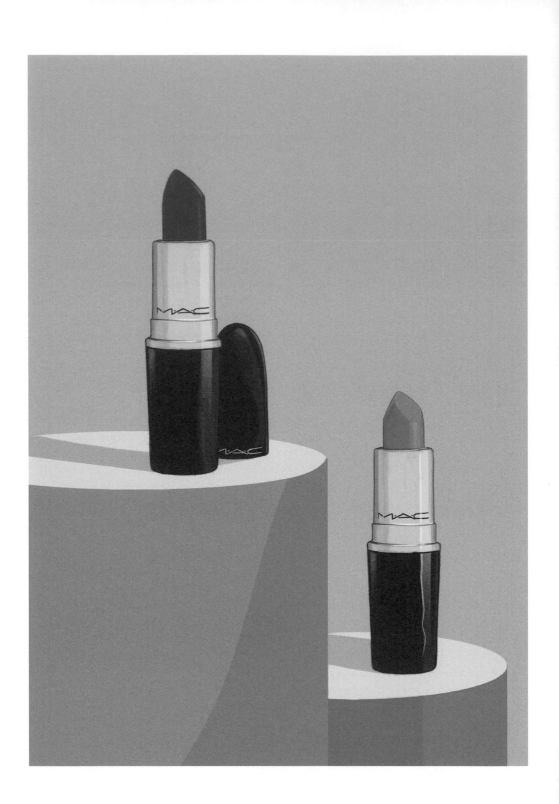

MAC
Lip Colours

I do not know where to begin with MAC's plethora of lip colours, textures, finishes... it's exhausting; it's a minefield. But it's a good one; a brilliant one, in fact. Because nowhere else can you get a more extensive range of pigments for your lips. The most popular, of course, is Ruby Woo, which is quite possibly the best-selling red lipstick in the world. I have yet to come across a woman who doesn't know or hasn't worn Ruby Woo. It's one of those colours you can spot a mile away. A deep bluey, superbly matte red lipstick that is universally flattering. If you haven't heard about it (have you been in a coma?), this is the red that suits everyone. If you are looking for a pinky red (something of a lifelong search for me – I don't want Pepto-Bismol or something that veers into the purple territory), then Relentlessly Red is perfection. And then there are nudes that actually look like 'our nude': Bronx is great. However, there is a range from which to choose, because, of course, people of colour come in all colours. (Quick! Someone tell the beauty industry!)

If you prefer liquids, which, more and more, I am gravitating towards, the **Retro Matte Liquid Lipcolour** range is phenomenal. So Me is a beautiful 'nude'. For a bright red, it's hard to beat Fashion Legacy, and if you prefer a deep pink, then To Matte With Love will light your fire. The thing with MAC is that it is not like most high-level cosmetics. Most of the big brands you see are all manufactured in the same factories around the world. MAC, on the other hand, has a secret formulation that cannot be replicated, meaning you will not find anything like it anywhere else. And that's great. The other thing with a number of MAC's matte lipsticks, however, is that they are notoriously drying; yet we keep buying them, not because we are all suckers, but because the colour pay-off is second to none. The solution? Get their **Prep + Prime Lip**, a colourless, oil-free, fragrance-free stick that you use before applying your lipstick. It is super hydrating and stops your lips from feeling like they are wearing a shield of liquid concrete.

FENTY BEAUTY
Stunna Lip Paint

Despite the hype around the Fenty Beauty foundations that undoubtedly were a game changer, it was the lip colour I was most interested in trying. Changing your foundation is like deciding to get married. It takes a whole lot of thought and commitment, and, of course, there is also something quite terrifying about it. Trying a lipstick, however, feels less so. Most women, like me, are quite breezily promiscuous with their lipsticks. If you are not, you should try it some time, it's fun. With this mantra in mind, I immediately made a beeline for Stunna Lip Paint in Uncensored. It is the shining bright-red liquid lipstick that comes in a glass bottle with a pointy pyramid-shaped top. The red paint (that description is appropriate) inside is without a doubt one of the very best liquid mattes and reds I have ever tried. Ever. It is phenomenal, imparting a pigment so quickly and gloriously that you forgive the slightly watery texture pretty much straight away. The doe-foot-ended wand is precise enough to make application a doddle, and one strike gives you all the colour you need. You can, of course, layer it, but why waste product and time when you don't need to? The colour has 12 hours' wear and is pretty much weightless on your lips, so you forget you have it on. And, best of all, it does not crack. The only issue is that, when applying, it is very difficult not to get it on your teeth, so do a quick check of those before leaving the house. Annoying but relatively inconsequential when you consider the merits of this product. It is truly amazing. Or, in Rihanna's inimitable words, this lip paint is 'One. Bad. Bitch.'

CHARLOTTE TILBURY
Hollywood Lips

I am a bright-lippie girl, which is something I never thought I would ever be. Like so many women of colour, I have very full lips. (Ironically, I am always sent lip-plumping products. Depending on my mood that moment, it makes me laugh or sigh.) Anyway, as a young girl and woman, I started off being very self-conscious about the size of my lips. There had been a few 'comments' thrown my way over the years. Rubber Lips/Tyre Lips/Why do you need armbands in the pool, surely your lips will help you float? Then, of course, there were the sniggering sexual comments, always unwanted. Invariably, you start doing whatever is necessary not to draw attention to them. And so, for a long time, I stuck to a mainly colourless gloss.

As my confidence as a woman grew, however, I started to dip my toe – well, my lips – into colour. I delved into muted pinks, because they were a little safe, although not necessarily successful. So many make-up brands never consider how pink translates on someone with quite dark lip pigment; not everyone's lips are naturally rosy pink. As I grew in years I became intrigued at the idea of finding my perfect red. I heard everyone has a red (it's true by the way), and so began my love of

brights. It is face lifting, confidence giving, ass kicking and just a complete delight wearing bright lipsticks. I celebrate my lips now. Not because they are big, but simply because they are mine, and that's enough.

There are still days, however, when I don't want to wear brights. But that's no longer because I am hiding. Sometimes it is just about a mood or being appropriate. I love juxtaposition; if I'm wearing a bright printed dress, I might want to counteract it with muted make-up, so I don't look like a human kaleidoscope. Then funerals; alas, I've been to a few. Wearing a punchy bright lip to one of those, well, you may as well go in dancing. The point is, there are days I want a muted, nude shade, which can be trickier to find than you'd think. Nonetheless, there is one, from Charlotte Tilbury's Hollywood Lips range, that is super modern, creamy and matte. As it is infused with beeswax, hyaluronic acid and sea lavender, it is not drying and doesn't cake. It is incredibly long wearing; I need never reapply during the day. There are a number of shades in the range, but the one I love is a nude pink that totally chimes with a darker skin tone. This shade's name? Show Girl. Yes, I thought you'd approve.

LIME CRIME
Matte Velvetines
Lipstick

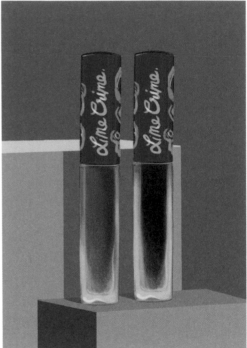

I must say the first thing I thought when I saw this is how much I disliked the packaging. I'm not saying everything should be an austere, pared-down ode to minimalism. Nor am I saying it should be all gold, shiny and the epitome of old-school luxury. It should just look … nice. Maybe it's those weird stencilled-looking flowers that do the range a disservice, because, on looks alone, I wouldn't take this seriously (there is something infantile about it), but, on performance, it smashes it. This brand, for those who haven't heard of it, is the original social-network brand that has weathered numerous storms (too many to go into) to become one of the coolest, cult, digital-first beauty brands.

Their Matte Velvetines range is known for being a pioneer in the liquid-lipstick movement, and they are still very much one of the best. The formulation is a creamy suede matte finish, which is the best. As it is pumped full of skin-nourishing ingredients, it feels comfortable on the lips and doesn't budge. The range of colours available is wide-ranging. The brights, particularly, are notable; Pink Velvet surely must be the ultimate pink. You also have left-of-centre shades, such as Black Velvet (for the Goth inspired – each to their own), Cement (a chic grey) and a deep purply plum called Fetish. They are all infused with vanilla, which I find slightly off-putting (for me, vanilla belongs in cakes, ice cream and milkshakes; not in beauty products). All the same, you might love it. Beyond that, the products are beautifully textured and brilliantly priced. The impressive delivery of pigment also showcases a quality that goes beyond that of other more expensive and well-known beauty brands. Just don't be put off by the strange-looking roses.

KEVYN AUCOIN
The Molten Lip Color: Molten Matte/Molten Gems/ Molten Metals

I am an Aucoin evangelist; beauty editors know and love the brand, but most people don't even know how to pronounce the name (it is R KWAN, by the way). It was founded by the late, legendary make-up artist of the same name, the man who paved the way for the likes of the influential British make-up artist Pat McGrath MBE, worked on numerous *Vogue* covers and famous names, and is largely credited as the man who invented modern make-up. In many ways, considering how influential Aucoin was/ is, it still surprises me how under the radar (for most people) the brand that takes his name is. Particularly as it is superb. Their Molten Matte liquid colours are worth a special mention. Every time I wear one, regardless of whether it is Julia (the bright orangey red) or Tori (a muted pinky nude), I get people asking, 'What is that?' (in the good way, not with a horrified face). They are the creamiest, smoothest mattes, long lasting and transfer resistant, and they don't dry the lips (thank you, camellia oil and vitamin E). If you are not a matte fan, there are also glossy (Molten Gems) and metallic (Molten Metals) ranges. The colourways are not particularly extensive, but they are all exceptionally strong.

Now, I don't know for how long you keep your lip colours, but they have a shelf life. How you store them, and general usage, will affect this. I had one for a few months, and then, one day, I opened it, and it smelt a little off (I'm trying to keep it cute and be diplomatic here). I realised I had left it in the sun and, additionally, that it wasn't quite closed all the way. So, my advice is to keep it closed, keep it clean and keep it out of the sun. It's an ethos that could probably serve us well in many areas of life.

STILA
Stay All Day®
Liquid Lipstick

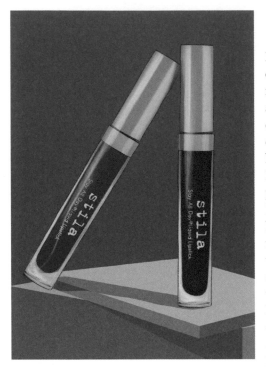

Fun Fact – you know that kick-ass bright-red lipcolour the US Congresswoman Alexandria Ocasio-Cortez sports? It's Stila Stay All Day® Liquid Lipstick in Beso. Ask any beauty aficionado about their most loved make-up products, Stila will be lurking in there somewhere. It was one of my go-to brands for lip colour for years, until it disappeared for a little while and then came back bigger and better. The thing is, the market has changed.

Brands have the problem of too much competition; it has become more and more difficult to get your voice heard and continue to be heard. As a result, as consumers, we have the quite nice problem of too much choice and the cacophony of launches makes it tricky to stay loyal. For lip colour, however, don't let Stila pass you by. The Stay All Day® Liquid Lipstick is just divine. It is a good entry-level matte for people who are still on the fence about them. It's not the kind of matte that is so powdery, opaque and devoid of all human life – or so intensely pigmented that you need a day just to get the first layer off. No, this is softly-softly stuff. It is deceiving because it looks like it could be a gloss. It has emollients such as vitamin E and avocado oil, which hydrate the lips beautifully, but the finish is matte. although in a wearable, non-intimidating way. The majority of the colour range (thirty-two at last count) is suitable for darker skin tones. It has about six hours' wear before reapplication is necessary, which is not bad at all. But unless I have lost my grasp of the English language it is not quite 'Stay All Day'. I don't suppose 'Stays on for 25 per cent of the Day' has quite the same ring.

CHANEL
Rouge Allure Luminous Intense Lip Colour

The quality of this lipstick is frankly beyond reproach. Among the many Chanel lipsticks, as the name suggests, this one has a luminosity, with none of the gloopy feeling of a full-on gloss. The sweet almond oil ingredient allows it to glide on effortlessly and feels so utterly comfortable that if you applied it in the dark, you'd swear you were wearing a balm. While I personally love the opaque density you get from an unapologetic vibrant matte, I know many find it tricky to wear: this texture offers a softer finish without sacrificing on an intense colour pay-off. Outstandingly, it can also be applied in a single stroke, making it undoubtedly the quickest, easiest lipstick I have ever used. At last count there were 24 shades in the range and I would say the majority of those will suit darker skin tones and lips, which most lip colour ranges do not consider. My favourites – which I like to wear with a lip liner for more definition – include Rouge Noir, a deep rich plum, Rouge Rebelle, a suits-everyone red (if you prefer a more understated red, try Incantevole) and Vibrante, a bright orange that is far more wearable than the bullet suggests. Shallow as it sounds, it would also be remiss of me not to mention the striking gold and black casing, which makes a magnetic 'click' sound when you open and close it. That sound (which, trust me, never gets old), is the sound of chic.

NARS
Powermatte
Lip Pigment

This is in a class of its own, which is classic NARS, to be honest. The brand just does things a bit differently, from the names of products (usually subversive and/ or a nod to popular culture) to aesthetics (the dense matte black with white writing is instantly recognisable). Everything is done on its own terms, regardless of how the industry is swaying. Once you begin using Powermatte, I predict it will remain part of your lipstick repertoire. The liquid has the lightness of a watercolour, and pigment that, on a scale of intensity, is like shopping in IKEA on a weekend. But unlike that divorce-inducing shopping experience, this is a positive intensity. It is a one-stroke, totally opaque swatch of colour for the lips. If you've come here for barely there colour, re-route. The wand has been described as doe-foot-shaped, but unless these animals have lots of different types of feet, I wouldn't call this that. Instead, it's a slightly curved triangle – still with a pointy top but softened and slightly flattened down the sides. In any case, it is a very effective applicator. This intense ink for lips doesn't dry down to a dead crisp. Instead your lips are still comfortable and flexible (you can move them, yay!), and they feel weightless. It doesn't transfer, and it lasts all day (and night, presumably; yes, it is that 'unbudgeable'). The range of colours available is an utter treasure trove. There are twenty-five of them, and every one is suitable for darker skins. If you want to go red/pink, try Don't Stop (a geranium red), You're No Good (a reddish pink) or Light My Fire (an orangey red) which are all conversation starters. For nudes, Just What I Needed is perfection, which seems a fitting note on which to end.

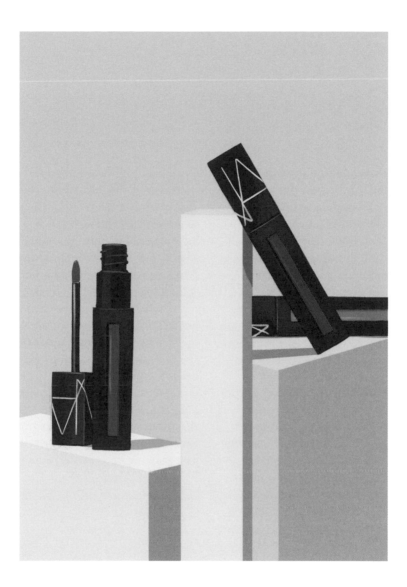

BOBBI BROWN
Matte Art Stick

One of the things I have loved most about writing this book is how much it has re-established my relationships with some of my loved ones. It's like a family reunion. A good family reunion. Not the one that ends in shouting, tears and doors slamming. This lipstick in a pencil is an old favourite that recently made its way back into my life. Anyone who loves simplicity with a bit of edge and a bit of fun will adore this. This is the sort of thing Bobbi Brown does so exquisitely. The brand speaks to every woman; it creates make-up for your everyday life but not in a way where practicality becomes a curse word. The Art Stick is literally a crayon for the lips. And, get this, each one even comes with a massive sharpener, which the child in me goes totally giddy over. The actual texture of the Art Stick feels like a lipstick but not in a shiny or sticky way. It just feels comfortable, almost like a balm. Interestingly, however, the finish is a comfortable matte. Genius. The pigment imparted is equally something to write home about. While it is fine to have something quite stiff and opaque that looks like it has been created via Artificial Intelligence, sometimes you want something like this, that is less rigid and more real. It has been enriched with shea butter (hence the wonderful feel on the lips), and it comes in a range of colours; the Rose Brown is an amazing nude. The brights, Harlow Red, Hot Pink and Sunset Orange, are epic. It is not a huge range, but I think you'll find all you need to form the basis of your lipstick wardrobe. It is excellent value, and unless you are using it as a chewing stick, it will last a while.

REVLON
Ultra HD Matte Lipcolor™

While I know that the quality and breadth of the high street/mass brands that incorporate the needs of darker skin tones have evolved over the years, I still don't automatically consider them a go-to. I guess it is a combination of things. As you get older you do steer towards brands that feel and look a bit more grown-up. Then there are the marks that certain experiences leave on you, which are difficult to erase. I still recall going into chemists and not finding things that worked on me – from lipsticks through foundations to something as basic as an eyeliner. It was always the same: the pigments and undertones were never deep enough, and I stopped bothering. I am more likely to buy a cheap eyeliner in a black hair-and-beauty store than from a chemist. The problem with giving up on the mass brands is that, invariably, you miss out on certain gems, such as this wonderful lip colour. I didn't find it myself (I had stopped looking); I happened across it when it was sent to me at *Vogue*. I was immediately drawn to the nude-ish shades (never mind finding the perfect reds, I've been on the hunt for a black-girl nude for a long time). It said it was matte, and I just look less like I've been in a time warp when I wear mattes, so I tried it. It was amazing. I had expected it to be, at best, passable. But it's a goodie. It has a lightweight, creamy, non-waxy texture that is slightly pasty but not unyieldingly so. It feels moisturising and velvety; perfect for those who want a lipstick that is neither shiny nor densely matte. This lies somewhere in between. The pigment cannot be compared to the more impactful finishes you get from some of the beauty industry's powerhouses, but it is an easy and cheap way to wear matte. You know what? It's not half bad.

Before bed, g
your lips wit
toothbrush a
balm. Your l
go on more s
the morning

ntly scrub
a soft
d apply lip
stick will
noothly in

MAC
Lip Pencils

I'll be totally honest here. I don't really bother much with other lip pencils as I am so insanely satisfied with what MAC has to offer that I don't see the point of looking elsewhere. It's like having a Michelin-starred chef cooking your daily meals at home and then visiting restaurants with lesser quality dishes. Curiosity may get the better of some, but the smart cookie will always come back home. We should all be that smart cookie. Sharp, pointy and solid, this pencil might look like any other pencil, but that's where the similarities end. You'd be forgiven for thinking the nib might be dry and drag when applying – it does look intimidatingly hard – but in fact, the creamy texture moves easily across the lips, meaning it doesn't take any type of skill to get that really crisp line which blends in seamlessly with your lipstick. The colours are also divine. Cherry and Ruby Woo, of course, are incredible reds. Currant is a lovely burgundy, Mahogany and Chestnut are great browns, Chilli, a very universal brick red if you want to go all out, and Talking Points is the perfect electric pink. Lip liners fell out of favour for a while but there is no substitute for getting that sharp, professional finish which they afford. This liner helps your lip colour go the extra mile, makes thinner lips look fuller and lasts an absolute age. In short, it gives you everything you could need in a lip pencil. Why on earth would you look elsewhere?

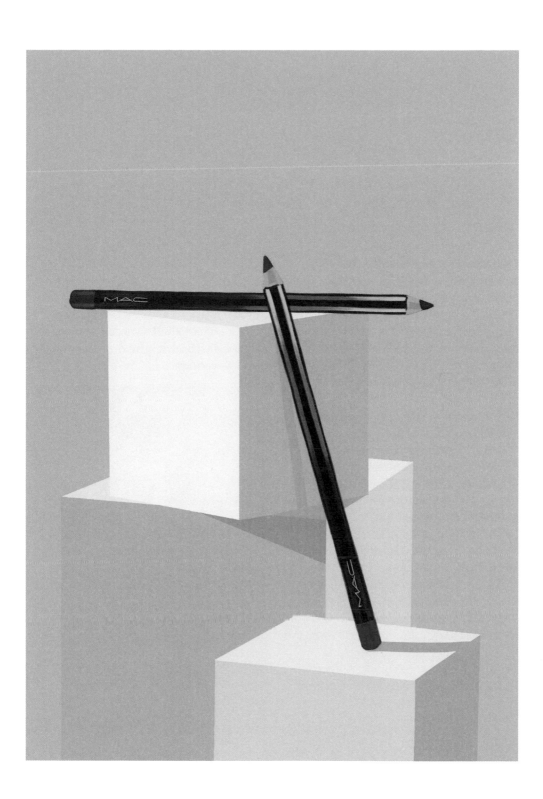

BOURJOIS
Rouge Velvet
The Lipstick

This Bourjois number falls into that wonderful new lipstick finish that brands are starting to tap into: velvet. Velvets are ideal for those who don't quite fancy the powdery density you get with a true matte, but desire pigment delivery with a silky, soft and – well – velvety finish. A large proportion of lipsticks that fit neither in the matte nor gloss departments have a no-man's-land formulation which either gives you a cheap finish or makes you look stuck in the 80s. This lipstick, however, delivers a punchy colour pay-off, supple lips and minimal reapplication. I also love the fact the opaque tube mimics the colour of the lipstick – a basic but brilliant touch which makes it easier to find in a sea of random stuff that has floated to the bottom of your bag (let's not even start on the wrinkle-inducing squint-fest you adopt just to read the teeny printed name). So bravo Bourjois, I'm impressed. The selection of colours for darker skin tones isn't extensive but what it does have is strong. I like 10, Magni-Fig, a purply pink, 11, Berry Formidable, which reminds me a little of Revlon's classic Black Cherry but not as dark, and 21, Grande Roux, a wonderfully flattering brick orange. For those sold on a brown lipstick there's 25, Maca'Brown. I might be yet to find someone who looks better with a brown lipstick on, but hey, it's a free country.

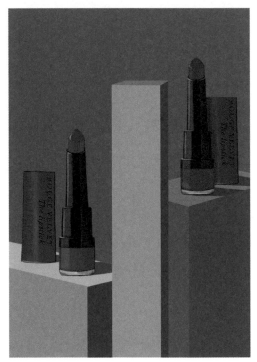

REVLON
Super Lustrous™
Lipstick

This lipstick has been around for decades, hence its strapline, 'The World's Most Iconic Lipstick'. Some may agree, others may see it as an exercise in exaggeration, but what everyone will hopefully agree on is that this is a beautifully formulated, highly pigmented and incredibly moisturising lipstick (cheers, avocado oil and vitamin E) which as far as high-street lipsticks go, is utterly faultless. Unlike many crème lipsticks in that category, it is not too shiny or sticky and it stays the course of the day. My personal standout shades include: Naughty Plum, which isn't actually a plum but more a brownish grape colour which translates into a brilliant nude for darker skin tones; Black Cherry, a sumptuous dark blood-red, is a modern classic; Fire & Ice, a bright vibrant red that may frighten wallflowers but is fabulous for the bold. Bombshell Red is that elusive, 'all-inclusive' red shade that looks good on pretty much everyone. For those who prefer a bold pink, Cherries in the Snow is right on the money. Sadly, the same can't be said for the packaging. The issue is that each lipstick comes wrapped in cellophane, and in many cases, there's also a coded sticker on the case, which is a pain to remove. That said, there is so much that Revlon are getting right; not least their representation of women of colour in their advertising, including models Adwoa Aboah, Achok Majak and Imaan Hammam all prominently fronting the 2018 'Live Boldly' campaign. A huge plus is the high quality of their lipsticks. So I'm willing to forgive the packaging missteps (in the hope it will be rectified) and simply enjoy this high street hero. I suggest you do the same.

CHANEL
Rouge Allure Liquid Powder Matte Lip Colour Blurred Effect

I have to say, the name of this product is slightly misleading. First, I thought it would literally be a powder that turns into a liquid. Then I assumed perhaps it was the finishing; maybe that would be super powdery, so there would be a high potential of it drying like Lottabody Setting Lotion. Back in the 1990s, that thing was hardcore; if you set your hair with it, not even a hurricane could pass through. Anyway, I was wrong on all counts. This creamy matte leaves lips soft and comfortable. And the finish is powdery. Surely an oxymoron? Well, whatever they have done in Chanel Towers, they have done right, because the formulation works. It uses an innovative technique to combine softening oils and highly pigmented shades in a way that leaves a velvety powdery finish that feels like silk. Beautiful and clever. The packaging and the application are also quite chic and innovative but very different for Chanel. It's what you imagine Chanel for a younger but still discerning audience would look like. Encased in a squeezy rubber tube, the top is a padded doe-footed-shaped (yes, that again) piece of foam. You squeeze and literally paint your mouth with it. There aren't many shades but, amazingly, due to the richness of pigment, I think they could all work on darker skin tones. My personal favourite shades are Invincible (a glorious red) and Bittersweet (an utterly sumptuous plum). I would advise prudence when squeezing to avoid waste. The finish is a blurred stain; for a more defined pout, I would recommend a lip liner. Anyone who has normally avoided mattes for fear of dryness will love this – there were times in the day I would forget and think I was wearing a balm, because it feels that comfortable. If you are the kind of girl who loves high-drama heavily pigmented opaque lipsticks that do not shift, consider this your off-duty alternative. But, of course, remember: this is Chanel, even dress-down days are fabulous.

CLINIQUE
Chubby Stick™ Moisturizing Lip Colour Balm

These chunky sticks are reminiscent of crayons, a nostalgia factor which I'm sure has been part of this best-seller's appeal. But aside from that, the success of this lip balm boils down to the fact that, quite simply, it works. Enriched with various oils, vitamin E, mango and shea butters, the ingredients are not so different to those found in many other lip balms, but what has kept this a cult product is its clever formulation. Unlike many other lip balms that either refuse to go beyond surface level or, ironically, make your lips drier, so you have to keep reapplying, this balmy texture delivers serious moisture, relieving cracked lips pretty much instantly without feeling greasy or heavy. Available in 16 natural tints across all shades, you get a pop of colour and shine, albeit one that is sheer and lightweight, so those with a penchant for deeper pigments may prefer the 'intense' options. I love a good colour payoff but on those mornings when you're taking the dog for a walk at 7am and can barely keep your eyes open, let alone swipe your lips with a pillar-box red, these balms rise to the occasion. They are a breeze to use – you famously don't need a mirror to apply, inexpensive and don't need sharpening (just swivel up). They are not so great when you desperately need a writing implement and it's the only thing to hand, but they will give you enviably soft lips.

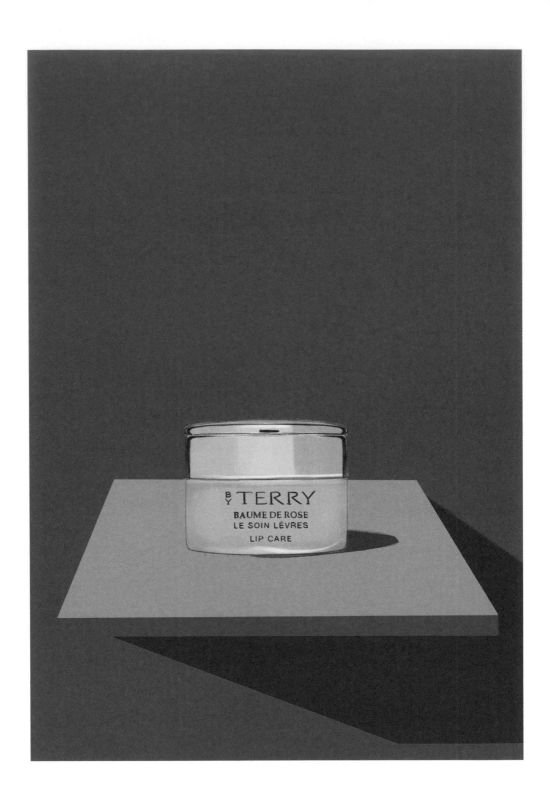

BY TERRY
Baume de Rose

Yes, I know, it is madly expensive. No, honestly, I haven't gone mad. The founder of the brand, Terry De Gunzburg is famed for the way she cleverly fuses make-up and skincare, but not in that half-assed way that some brands do. No, she absolutely goes all in, which is why, in many ways, to think of this as just a lip balm would be somewhat insulting. You can't compare it to Vaseline, that would be like saying Beyoncé and the woman who has been leading karaoke at the local pub for the past 12 years are both singers. Equally, you cannot compare this to other lip balms. There are lip balms and then there is this. It is a magical concoction that has been formulated with vitamin E, shea butter, antioxidants, ceramides (help the skin retain moisture), rose flower wax and pastel oil. It is a winning formula that has a cult following of beauty editors and A-listers, and it is totally worthy of its high status. This slightly thick (and, yes, balmy), textured product is scented with rose and glides on beautifully without leaving shine, which is great. I don't understand lip balms that leave you shiny. If I want a shine, I'll get a gloss. Also, Baume de Rose is the first lip balm I have used that hasn't had a counterproductive effect and made my lips drier than they were before. It is effective on cuticles, on hands and even on children. My eldest was born incredibly prematurely, and after spending months in the intensive-care unit his skin began to get really irritated. Everything the doctors suggested and prescribed did not work. This lip balm, on the other hand, did. Yes, it is an expensive lip balm. But, in reality, it is so much more than that.

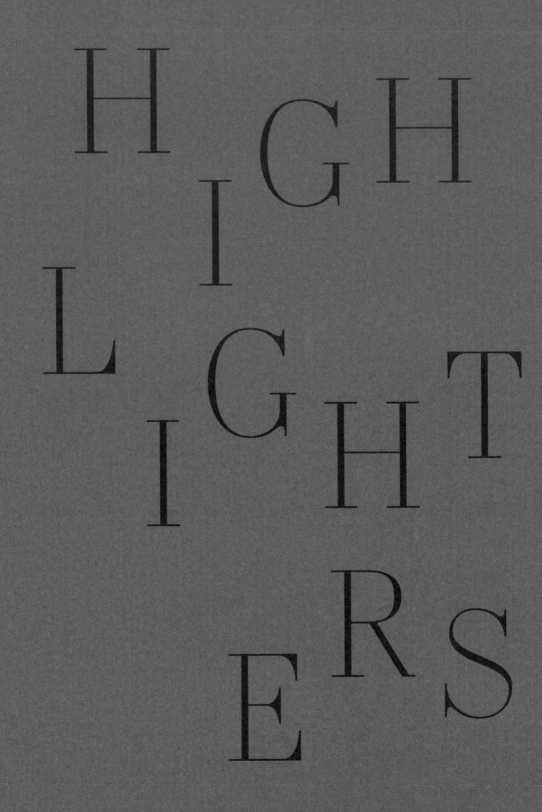

HIGHLIGHTERS

THINGS TO NOTE...

The purpose of a highlighter is
to highlight key parts of your face –
tops of cheeks and brow bones – so
they look glorious when you hit the
light. If appropriate, mix it in with
foundation. Rich tones, such as golds,
coppers and bronzes, are warmer and
more complementary on our skin
tones; silvery tones, not so much.
Avoid dusting highlighter all over your
face – unless you're auditioning for
a role in a futuristic film, I wouldn't
recommend it.

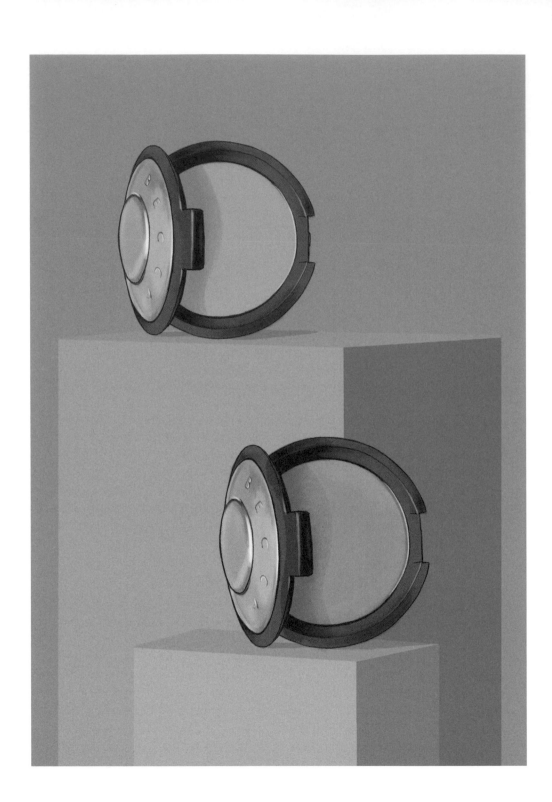

BECCA
Shimmering Skin Perfector® Liquid Highlighter/Pressed Highlighter

So, I've said this before: I have an imaginary beauty category called 'I'd drink it if I could'. This product, in its various forms, hovers somewhere at the number-one spot (there are a few jostling at number one, because I'm generous like that). To put it bluntly, this highlighter is magnificent. It comes in different textures – the liquid version has been described on numerous occasions as soft focus in a bottle. And that is right. I use Topaz on a daily basis because it fools people into thinking you have the best skin in the world. Why it works is threefold.

It is glossy (leaving you with a dewy finish); it is the right shade of gold (more golden-coppery gold; not so gold you look like the dead woman in *Goldfinger*), and it has no glitter in it (which would look ridiculous if you go anywhere you want to be taken seriously; no, it shouldn't matter, but it does). Then there are all the skin benefits. It is oozing with antioxidants to protect your skin from free radicals, and it also includes witch hazel (for inflammation) as well as various hydrating ingredients to boost moisture levels in the skin. It gives you skin an unbelievably illuminated and blurred to perfection finish that it is near impossible not to become addicted to.

I use this in my foundation daily. I mix them together, then apply that, as you would a serum – I don't tend to bother with a brush. Immediately, my face comes alive. I do find it is one of the few highlighters I can use without bits of shimmery stuff getting caught in pockets of my skin – it blends well and leaves your skin blurred, but dewy, and perfected. another bonus is the bottle which lasts a long time because you only need a teeny single pump.

So far I have been referring to the liquid version. If you prefer a more powdered finish, then it stands to reason that the pressed version is best (Chocolate Geode is great for even deeper skin tones). It also enables you to target specific areas, such as the tops of the cheekbones. You will need to apply this using a brush, but if you are excessive, it is more likely to end in disaster; hence, for something more malleable, the liquid is your best bet. It also used to come in a 'poured' version, a hybrid of the liquid and the powder. Annoyingly, they discontinued it. Thankfully, they left us with the best liquid highlighter in the world. Just try not to drink it.

MAC
Strobe Cream

I remember when the Strobe Cream first came out. Well, actually, I don't know if it was when it first came out – it could be when I first discovered it. Needless to say, I didn't really know what to do with it. I remember a friend saying you could put some on a brush and dot it on the inside corners of your eyes because 'it's what all the celebrities do'. And, of course, everyone's top priority in life should be to look like a celebrity, otherwise why are you still breathing? Still, I followed her advice. My 'technique' wasn't great, so I just looked like something had gone terribly wrong, and I had 'sleep' in my eyes. It also made my eyes weep. Then I thought perhaps I should just use it all over. I did, and I looked like a very unhappy robot. These days, however, I know that Strobe Cream was/is a highlighter. It was just way before its time. Look closer, though, and you will see that it is so much more than a traditional highlighter. This silky, radiance-inducing iridescent cream is fused with green tea and various vitamins to awaken and hydrate the skin. Back then the only shade it came in was sheeny silver. It now also comes in various shades; the pink is gloriously warm on darker skin tones. You can mix this in with your foundation, or, if you prefer a matte finish, just use it in specific areas to stop skin from looking flat (alternatively, mix it with a highlighting powder). For everyone else, say hello to the original dewy skin, darling.

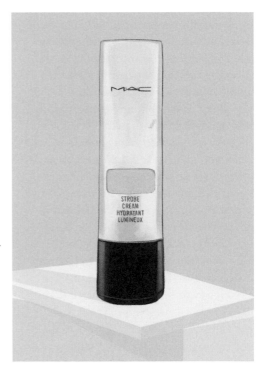

FENTY BEAUTY
Killawatt Freestyle Highlighter

Every time I fall in love with new products, I have a habit of starting a new make-up bag to accommodate them. It's not that I never revisit the old bag, I do from time to time, but then, after a while, I've built up something of a harem of new make-up bags that I just can't keep up. I imagine this is how a bigamist must feel. Anyway, every so often you simply change your make-up bag, because you have no choice. Like when your Killawatt highlighter compact completely smashes to smithereens in it. If anyone knows this highlighter, you will feel my pain. It is a beautiful, intensely, pigmented cream–powder illuminiser. It is one of the few you can use on top of your base without it disappearing into the ether because your foundation shade just swallows it up (which is why it's rare for me to recommend a cream blush). Due to the formulation, I feel this product is easily one of the absolute best in the entire Fenty Beauty collection. You'd be hard pushed to find anything in this no-glitter finish that has such an impressive delivery of pigment and goes on so exquisitely. It comes in various shades: Trophy Wife (an intense gold) is probably the most famous. Ginger Binge–Moscow Mule (a muted pinky burgundy duo) are the two most flattering shades on darker skin tones. It is best applied with a brush but do exercise caution. I can always tell the overexcited coterie of people who have recently invested in a Fenty highlighter and have taken the bull-in-a-china-shop approach. If the world suddenly lost its light, they would be human torches. It's a terrifying look. As is the sight of it smashed in your make-up bag. Intense does not even begin to cut it.

NARS
The Multiple/Light Sculpting Highlighting Powder/ Illuminator

If there were one brand I'd recommend as a one-stop shop for highlighters to suit all needs and levels of proficiency, I would recommend NARS. There is so much here to love. When The Multiple, which has become a best-selling cult product, was launched, the word highlighting wasn't even in popular make-up vernacular. This multi-use stick is a creamy formulation with shimmer (not glitter!) that can be used all over your face and even on your body. It is a beautifully silky cream formulation that is malleable and pretty much foolproof (if you put it on, and it doesn't look right, just blend it in with a brush). It stays put all day. The delivery of pigment to the skin is the perfect balance: great colour pay-off but not so intense that it masks the skin. As with all NARS products, the ranges are incredibly inclusive and there is a wide shade selection from which to choose. Na Pali Coast (a pinky bronze), one of my favourites, leaves a dewy golden glow on the skin.

If you want something to lift a matte foundation, the Light Sculpting Highlighting Powder is epic. St. Barths (a golden bronze) and Maldives (a rose bronze) are both glorious. They are created with a Seamless Glow Technology, which, on a basic level, is a crush of powders and pearls that leaves you with a glowy finish that feels like satin on the skin. Unlike most powders, it doesn't highlight imperfections or age skin, rather it makes your skin look more youthful and a million times better. This releases much more pigment than The Multiple and I would suggest only using it on certain points. If you use it all over, you'll look like a robot.

For something you can either mix into your foundation or even wear on its own, Illuminator takes some beating. It's a multifunctional iridescent boost for your face. Worn alone, it gives the skin a natural, beautiful glow, especially in the summer. When mixed with foundation, it will escalate your finish from good to amazing. The best shade for darker skin is Orgasm, a peachy pink with shimmer liquid that is inspired by the classic blush of the same name. But if you want to up the ante, try the Super Orgasm. The name speaks for itself; I'll say no more.

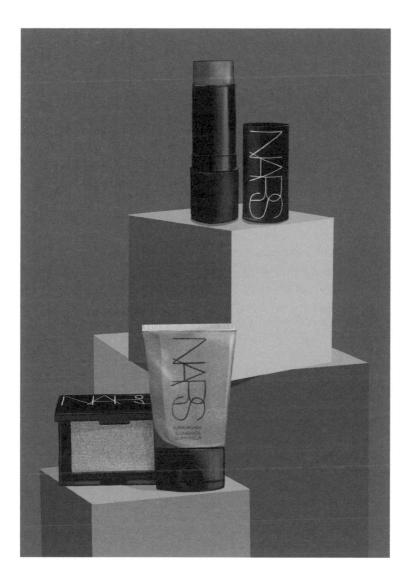

RMS
Beauty Contour
Bronze

One afternoon, I hung out with the force that is Rose-Marie Swift, veteran make-up artist (*Vogue, Harper's Bazaar, Allure, Louis Vuitton* and so forth) and founder of RMS Beauty. I've spent time with many brand founders who are so media trained they have the personality of a plank. With Rose-Marie, it's like being blindfolded and spun around in a wind tunnel. She is all consuming, funny, brilliant and outspoken. Even if you don't believe in her truths and theories (she has a lot to say about the state of the nations and the industry), it is certainly an experience you don't forget. Her line is just as uncompromising: it is non-toxic, natural but efficacious beauty. She has been a huge 'conscious beauty' proponent ever since a health scare caused her to look into symptoms she believed were caused by beauty products she had been using up until that point. Anyone who knows me knows that I have always been rather snitty about so-called natural beauty brands, because so many are not worth the time. This, on the other hand, is. If you are looking for a non-sparkly, slightly understated highlighter that is multi-tasking, more bronze than gold, super easy to use and highly unlikely to go wrong, then you've come to the right place. It is a beautifully formulated bronzer-highlighter hybrid with a slightly balmy texture that ushers you into happy-skin territory. It is super adaptable and buildable, but I wouldn't use it all over: it's too subtle and sheer to really stand out within your foundation. It is better off used in other ways. You can tap it on to the tops of your lids or your cheekbones, where it catches the light, or use it as a subtle contour. 'Subtle' is the objective word here. If you are looking for the Instagram-style contour that makes you look like an A1 model (I mean, why would you?), sorry, this is a highlighter for real life.

HUDA BEAUTY
3D Highlighting Palette

If you are a highlighter pro on the search for a one-stop shop to give you that no-filter-required Insta glow, this is your crack. If you are a highlighter novice, this might be your worst nightmare, because, for you, this is a palette of four colours, and four bits of instructions that may as well read: 'mammoth opportunity for things to go horribly wrong'. This, as you may have gathered, is not a highlighting kit I would recommend for beginners. Yes, there are directives on the inner lid of the palette: Prep, Set, Sculpt, Flush. However, unless you hate your life (I mean, you want to waste your life; sorry, I mean you spend your life watching millions of beauty vlogs), the instructions may as well be written in Aramaic (you wouldn't have a clue what to do with it). I would suggest first building your confidence with liquid/creamy highlighters. They are infinitely easier to navigate than powders and less likely to leave you with what might be mistaken for shimmery tribal marks.

For the smug pros who know their way around a highlighter with their eyes shut, these formulations are perfection. They are inspired by Huda's beauty hack of layering oil with powder. Despite them looking like straight-up powders, these are actually slightly creamy pearlescent bases, with the most intense colour pay-off. They have been infused with shea butter, so they blend seamlessly into skin; that is, they won't get stuck in and highlight your pores. The palettes come in a number of colour options but Bronze Sands (the perfect mix of coppers, bronzes and golds) is what I would recommend for darker skin tones. These are easily some of the best highlighters on the market: the undertones are on point, and they are guaranteed to give you the perfect 'lit-from-within' skin. But only if you know what you are doing.

COVER FX
Custom Enhancer Drops

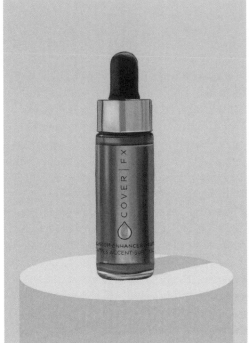

There are numerous beauty products that seem like the most normal thing to me. And then I step out of the bubble that exists in the beauty industry and onto social media, and I realise that IRL most human beings are utterly befuddled by highlighters. I totally get that. Use the right one in the wrong way, and your metallic face will spook your neighbours. Use the wrong one and, well, there is just no right way to use the wrong highlighter. If you would like to have a highlighted face (one that radiates an enviable luminous glow; not one that looks like it's on fire), the easiest way to achieve this is via a liquid highlighter. These drops, intensely pigmented illuminators, are genius. There are currently seven shades in the range: Halo (a holographic silver), Blossom (a soft pearlescent pink), Rose Gold (a pinkish bronze), Celestial (a glistening pearl), Moonlight (a shimmering beige), Sunlight (a glowing gold) and Candlelight, my favourite (a golden bronze). Cover FX is well known for its inclusive approach to make-up; amazingly, all the drops have been formulated to work across all skin tones. Just add a drop or two into your foundation or your skincare (be it serum or moisturiser) and apply to your face.

Hello, luminous sun-kissed skin. There are no glitter particles in this, just an elegant shimmer. The finish on your skin is entirely dependent on what you mix in with the drops. How highlighted you look hangs on how many drops you add. You can, of course, always dial up or down. But do remember: it is incredibly concentrated; if you finish it in under six months, you should be booked into rehab for highlighter addiction. Final piece of advice: the brand suggests also using it on its own. Unless you are a highlighter pro, I wouldn't.

MAC
Mineralize Skinfinish

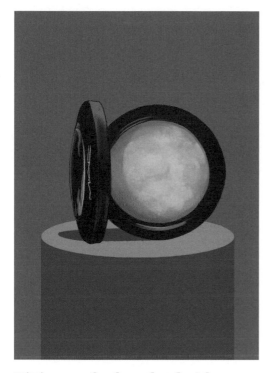

A velvety soft, luminous highlighting powder that features MAC's famed 77-Mineral Complex and vitamin E, it comes in six shades, although I tend to stick to Gold Deposit because it's the one I find most 'natural' on darker skin tones. Do, however, take the word 'natural' with a pinch of salt, because, honestly speaking, there is nothing particularly natural about it. This highlighter is so fiercely pigmented that if you get it on your favourite dress, read that frock its last rites and be done. If you are looking for something more natural, then you are better off going for a sheer gloss-based highlighter. The finely ground texture of this highlighter, along with its skin-loving ingredients, does mean that it blends beautifully. But the trick to success is down to application. If you use it on your brush, do a light sweep and dust it around your brow bone and the top of your cheekbones. For an awesome glow – and this is going to sound laborious but, trust me, it works – I'd advise you to scrape a teeny bit off the top and mix it with your foundation and then apply it to your face. It gives you the most exquisite sun-kissed finish. Whatever you do, resist the urge to brush it all over your face – you will look like an Oscar.

Hitting pan, for those that don't know, is when you use your powder/bronzer/blusher/eyeshadow so much, you reveal the metal of the container beneath the product. This highlighter, certainly in the last few years, is the only product I have ever hit pan with. When it got right down to the end, I was like a child who finishes off her ice cream and licks the bowl when she thinks no one is looking. That is how much I love it.

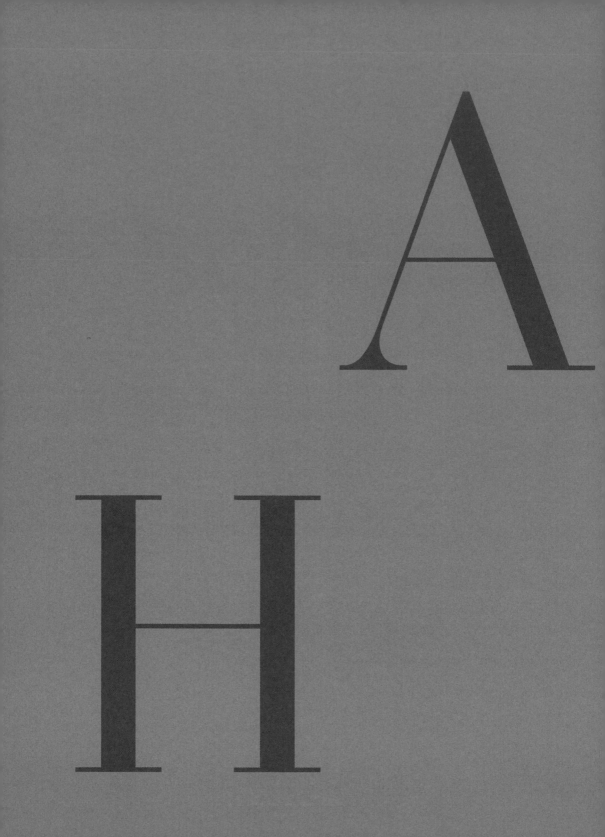

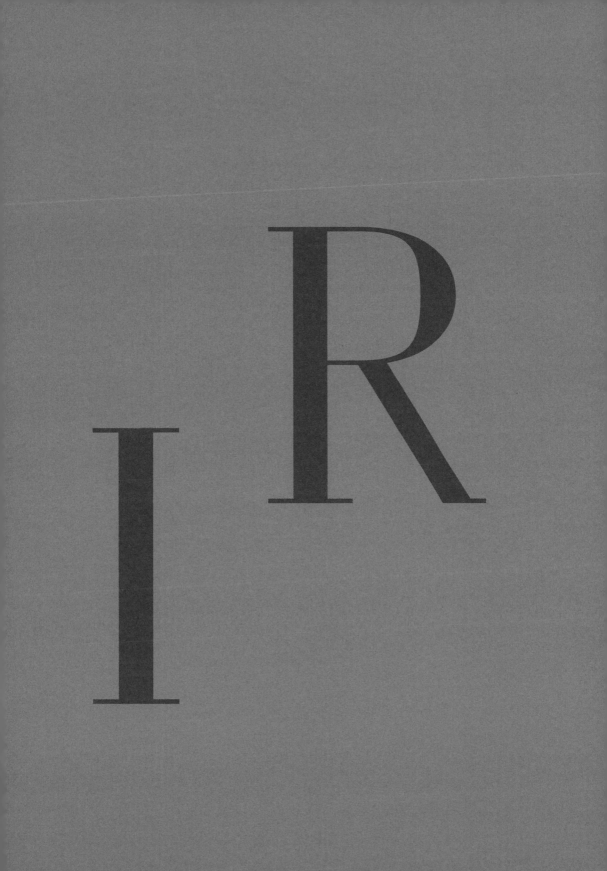

HAIR CARE

I receive certain emails from beauty PRs that cause me to do a lot of eye rolling. At least once a week, someone invites me to have a spray tan. While I'm not arrogant enough to think every PR in the industry knows who I am, we can all covertly stalk people on Instagram (you know you do), so surely sending such a badly targeted email is just lazy. Also, does Funmi Fetto sound like a Caucasian name to you?

I also get 'hair' emails. Some offer an appointment to come in to have my hair done, but then I look at their offering and realise they don't even have Afro/textured hair services. Then you get those who ask me to come in for an 'Express Blow-dry'. Does such a thing even exist in our hair vernacular? Express and Blow-dry (in the 'swishy hair' way they mean it) are not two words one associates with our hair. I don't even bother responding, because the way I see it, that email was not meant for me. And that's the problem right there. While many beauty brands are working hard to show the world just how inclusive they are, most mainstream hair brands are not even trying to cater for different hair types. I have attended numerous haircare launches, where the founders speak, without batting an eyelid, about how they have created a line that delivers 'beach waves' and 'you know, that cool, French-girl hair'. Sorry, darling, no, I don't know.

The mainstream hair industry is so wildly behind the curve, which, from a commercial perspective, is crazy, considering evidence shows women of colour spend up to eight times more on products than their Caucasian counterparts. So why does the industry ignore this? Is it racism? Or ignorance? I don't have the answer. What I do know is that while this section of the book celebrates some of my favorite hair products, the omission of a huge number of well-known brands is a damning indictment of mainstream haircare producers and their inability to truly embrace inclusivity. Specialist shops in areas with a high concentration of non-white residents shouldn't be the only places a black woman can find suitable hair products.

My choices are a mix of mainstream and niche brands (some you never would guess work well on textured hair) as well as some that are ubiquitous in any good 'black hair shop' which I love. This is the place I spend hours discovering random brands with hilarious names, superficially fragranced products, kitsch packaging and the hyperbolic promise of strands thicker than your ankles and hair so long you could sit on it. I relish it all. And I know so many women feel the same way because hair is such a thing for us: the history, the essays, the poetry, the features, the politics, the songs... And the plethora of textured-hair YouTube videos championing and slating products in equal measure. My hope is that you will fall in love with the following products, just as I have.

HAM
S A M
S O
P O S

THINGS TO NOTE...

Foam is not the enemy – it depends
with what else it is formulated with.
Moisture is your best friend, especially
if your hair is natural. Cheap does
not mean bad. Expensive doesn't
always mean better. Co-washes are
wonderfully gentle, conditioner-led
hair cleansers (what a mouthful), but,
at some point, you are still going to
need a shampoo. Nothing short of an
old-school cleanse is going to sort out a
month's worth of build-up.

IGK
Hot Girls Hydrating Shampoo

For the purpose of upholding what I hope is a reputation as a decent beauty editor, I end up trying a lot of things. Like this product. In normal circumstances, I would have completely bypassed IGK. Not for any terrible reason but as a brand it seems very much geared towards the 'cool' Insta-influencer, aspiring to that rock-and-roll/ beachy tousled hair and an irreverent attitude. These are the kind of girls who get a million likes for their posts about their kale supplements, green juices and vegan-everything life choices. All the things that make you feel more marginalised than ever. Nevertheless, I was attracted to the word 'hydrating' because I have long discovered it is the key to 'Happy Hair' (that's my non-discriminatory replacement term for 'Good Hair') and this shampoo is now a core and much-loved member of my hair repertoire. It really does what it says on the tin: it is an exquisite hydrator; one of the few hair products that claims to be 'suitable for all hair textures' and actually delivers on Afro hair. It smells really coconut-y but not in an oppressive way. I'm not even sure if it has coconut in it, but it does have vitamin E, built-in UV protection and litchi extract to protect hair from oxidative stress (which is when there is an imbalance between the free radicals that attack the body and the body's ability to fight back). It has no sulphate, which I know everyone is obsessed with eschewing (I'm still on the fence on that one); but unlike most sulphate-free shampoos it foams (Hurrah! I love foam!), and it cleans without stripping the hair. Best of all you can just about get away with using it without a conditioner – it makes your curls soft, frizz free, shiny and defined. The Dream.

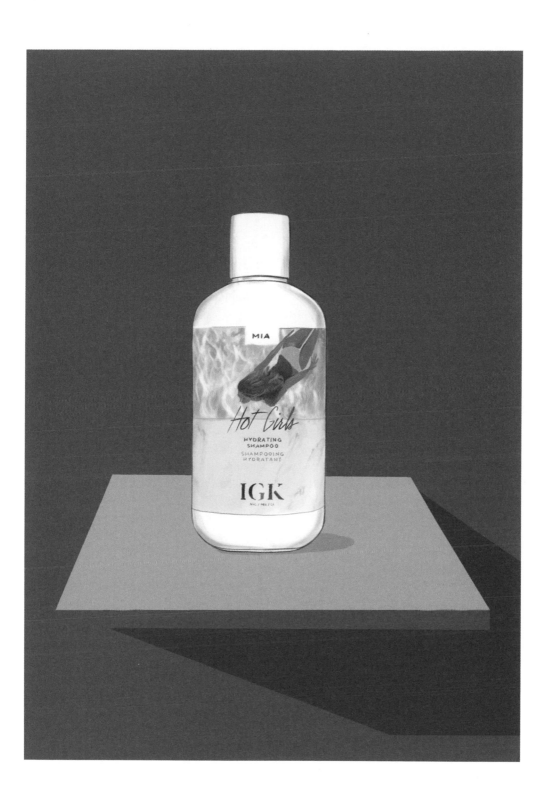

PANTENE
Gold Series Moisture Boost Shampoo

So, the first time I used this, I was blind-testing it. It was an off-white, foamy-looking thing that appeared suspiciously like a thick, expensive bubble bath. Aside from a teeny label that said 'shampoo' on it, there were no clues to exactly what it was. Like a willing, excited guinea pig, I used it and WOW. This shampoo is easily, and I don't say this lightly, one of the best I have used. It is infused with argan oil but, to be honest, that doesn't mean that much; I've come across lots of products with argan oil that make absolutely no difference to skin or hair. It's all about the formulation, and nowhere did this feel more evident and relevant than with this shampoo. You see, it contains sulphate. Yes, there you are, running for the hills. But here's the thing: the brouhaha around the evils of sulphate is misguided and misinformed. Speaking with the brilliant head scientist behind this product, a woman of colour with Afro hair, she explained that sulphate in and of itself is not bad. It is all about what you put with it. Sulphate is an ingredient that will have a negative or positive reaction based on the dosage and with what other ingredients it is formulated. It was fascinating to hear this, as everyone else seems scared to challenge the general consensus on this ingredient. While I am no science professor, however they have formulated this has hit the nail on the head. It has an immediate softening effect and makes detangling a cinch, and my hair feels intensely moisturised. And it was so cheap! Excuse my overzealous (ab)use of the exclamation mark, but, on this occasion, it is warranted, because I've experienced shampoos ten times the price that are nowhere near as good. Still, there is also a sulphate-free version. Whichever you choose, your hair will still thank you for it.

TEXTURE MY WAY®
Hydrate! Intensive Moisture Softening Shampoo

Can we please talk about the packaging?
Can we? I'm so sorry, but if it were down
to packaging alone, this definitely would
not make the cut. How many words, fonts
and lines need to be on the front of a
beauty product? How many? And why is
it SO green? It's so tiresome consistently
seeing products aimed at women of
colour looking as if they were put together
by someone with a bad case of design
diarrhoea. I just needed to get that off my
chest. Now, let's talk about the otherwise
fabulous product. It is infused with lots
of shea butter and various natural oils to
soften and add moisture. Which it does
really well, particularly on mixed-heritage
Afro-hair types (thicker, coily hair may feel
they need a bit more hydration). It cleans
brilliantly and quickly without stripping,
so hair is not left feeling like crackling.
Still, I wouldn't necessarily advise skipping
the conditioning step, but if you did, your
detangling process won't be as traumatic as
you might think. For all the wrong reasons,
I absolutely love the smell. Like so many
of the old-school products you discover
in 'ethnic' beauty-supply stores (which,
of course, is how I found this, among
a cacophony of products with equally
maddening packaging), the scent is overly
fruity, overly floral and overly fragranced
(and it also looks like yellow bubble bath).
So if you have a fragrance-free ethos,
this will freak you out, because, despite
being sulphate, paraben, mineral oil and
petroleum free, the scent is so hilariously
out of step with the current trend for
products that smell of air. Which says it's
either totally behind the curve or just a
beauty rebel doing its own thing and doing
it well. I like to think it's the latter.

SHU UEMURA
Art Of Hair Essence
Absolue Cleansing Milk

If co-washes were football clubs, this would be in the Premier League. It is just divine. But we shouldn't be surprised about that. I find many Japanese beauty products are pretty superior, and this one doesn't fall short. As with all the best products, I stumbled upon it by complete accident when I was sent the wrong product and then decided to try it anyway. I had no expectations – co-washes weren't really a thing at that point – and it blew my mind. The creamy, superluxe texture looks expensive (like an exorbitantly priced moisturiser you'd pick up in the Harrods Beauty Hall). It also smells expensive, and I discovered that the scent is structured in the same way you would a perfume, that is, in layers and notes, which here include grapefruit, green almond, camellia and velvety musks), making it so much more elevated than your average hair product. When you use it, your hair immediately begins to feel like melting butter. This is the magic of camellia oil. It comes from the hardy Camellia japonica tree, known for its strength and ability to survive in pretty much any situation. The oil protects the hair from drying out and leaves it supersoft, silky and detangled. Now, before we get too excited, there are a few caveats of which you should be aware. It foams, but it is ever so subtle, so a good compromise that will satisfy diehard foam-lovers and appease the anti-foam brigade. Then there's the issue of hair texture. When I first began using this, I was transitioning from chemically processed/relaxed hair to natural hair. At a time when the texture of my hair was a little bit ambiguous, this cleansing milk was a lifesaver. It made my hair feel much more uniform as opposed to highlighting the different textures; everything felt softer, shinier, and my curls began to take shape. Since going completely natural, however, I have found that while this still works, I definitely need much more product to get the same results – my hair is very thick; the texture somewhere between 4b and 4c. And if I have product build-up, it takes so much longer to cleanse the hair. Then there's the packaging. The squeezy tube is a pain – you have to exert a lot of pressure to get the product out (Shu Uemura, please can you just put the damn thing in a tub? If I want to exercise my biceps, I'll go the gym). Nevertheless, the hair-softening, curl-cleansing properties and the scent make this product special. There are co-cleansers, and then there's this incredible cleansing milk.

CHRISTOPHE ROBIN
Cleansing Purifying Scrub With Sea Salt

So many of us have been indoctrinated into thinking the old-school ritual of a hairdresser washing our hair like she or he has anger-management issues is the most natural thing in the world. In fact, when I have visited hair stylists who don't wash my hair with that level of intensity, I have always come away thinking my hair isn't quite clean enough. But that's a fallacy. It is possible to exfoliate your scalp and clean your hair without such misplaced zeal. This gritty-textured – literally, large sea-salt grains – citrus-scented, sweet-almond-oil scrub does that job perfectly. It will detox, cleanse and invigorate the scalp, swiftly, gently but incredibly effectively. It also gets the blood circulating, which, ultimately, means healthier hair growth. (If we spent half as much time, money and effort on our scalps as we do on our hair, we would see a huge difference.) This shampoo–scalp-treatment hybrid is a cult product for good reason. So how to use it? Well, like a shampoo. Sort of. Most shampoos will say you only need a pea-sized dollop to wash your hair.

They are talking rubbish. You always need more. But this one is correct in that regard. Any more than a teaspoon of the stuff, and you'll be drowning in the suds for months to come. Ah, yes, there is sulphate in this, and it foams. It's a robust and unapologetically foamy foam that sulphate-haters might take as a personal affront. If there is any consolation, it is paraben, silicone and colourant free. And it rids the hair of any chemical residue – hence its popularity as a post-colour, post-beach and post-pool wash, although I wouldn't use it daily. It is perfect if you have a lot of build-up due to braids and heavy-product use. And for people who think it is perfectly acceptable to only wash your hair quarterly (we won't judge; we just won't talk about that). If there is a con to this incredible cleanser, it's that it cleans, perhaps, a little too well. There are some shampoos you can get away with using and skipping the conditioner step. This is not one of them.

TRESEMMÉ
Moisture Rich Shampoo

Now it is an incredibly rare (read: non-existent) situation for me to buy my hair products in an everyday chemist or supermarket. The aisles that hold hair products in those outlets are pretty much dead to me. However, on a trip buying mundane necessities (because sometimes even a beauty editor has to buy exciting things like toilet cleaner), I spotted this bottle. It was huge – bigger than my head – it was half price, and it had the words MOISTURE written on it in big, fat letters. The great thing about experimenting with hair products is that it's not like skincare. Here, the damage is fairly limited; whatever goes wrong can more or less be remedied. (That is unless, of course, you stupidly decide to chemically process and dye your hair within the same hour. As you watch clumps of your hair fall into the bath, you will be so stunned your screams will leave your lips soundlessly. In a situation such as this, there is no remedy; you are, for want of a better word, stuffed. And, yes, I speak from experience.) So I went for it; I had nothing to lose. Worst-case scenario, it would turn out to be dire, and I'd just use it as a body wash (which is what I do with useless shampoos; if it's really shocking, I'll use it to clean the bath). I needn't have worried. This sweetly scented (not nauseatingly so) shampoo was marvellous. Immediately my parched hair felt like it had been given an injection of hydration. It is hugely moisturising – it has vitamin E in it – and really softens the hair; it also washes beautifully. Yes, it does foam, but it doesn't strip; so even for really dry hair, this is an absolute godsend – you'll find the texture of your curls softer, silkier and frizz free. It sounds trite, but a little really does go a long way. And seeing as the bottle I bought is the size of a dumb-bell, it'll be an eternity before I need to replace it.

FUNCTION OF BEAUTY
Bespoke Shampoo

Growing up I was terrible at science. These days I try to convince myself that I read *Scientific American* because it's just so wonderfully enjoyable, but the truth is I read it for work, and I still look at people who love science as I would someone with three heads. Nevertheless, the idea of being my own alchemist has always appealed; that is, mixing things up to suit my own preferences – clashing prints, red lips and green eyes, jam and butter – try it, it is epic. And I did go through a phase of making homemade beauty products but washing shea butter out of blenders quickly lost its appeal. Still, when I heard about Function of Beauty, a personalised haircare brand based in New York, I was all over it. The idea is that you go through a (quick) series of questions on hair texture, hair issues, hair goals and so on. You also choose your scent (or not) and the finishing colour (of the product, not your hair). And then, *voilà*, you have your very own cruelty-, sulphate- and paraben-free set of shampoo and conditioner. It also appeals to the aesthete in me – their minimalist logo as well as your name/initials are printed on the equally minimalist capsule-shaped bottles. Of course, there is nothing particularly novel about personalisation, and I'm sure if you searched long enough, you could absolutely find a specialist to create a hair product specifically for you. The difference is you'd probably need to sell your kidneys to afford it. The beauty here is the price, which while not high-street cheap, is a snip considering it is totally bespoke. Plus, you can arrange a standing order of sorts, so you receive a monthly or three-monthly delivery. There are downsides, though: it's not a quick buy as it can take up to 14 days to arrive. Also, it might require a couple of tryouts before you get the formulation exactly right. The first time I used this, I ticked the wrong hair goals (it was late, I was tired, I am human), and so the formulation was not exactly right for me. I also asked for a 'light' scent (it was too subtle), because I thought anything more intense would be heavy handed – like when you ask for a burger 'well done' and you get a lump of charcoal. But the question really is: does it work? The answer is: absolutely. And if it doesn't, well, it's probably the 'manufacturer's fault. And, in this case, that would be you.

AVEDA
Sun Care Hair And Body Cleanser

I have a strange relationship with multi-tasking products. On the one hand, I love the time-saving aspect of something that kills two birds with one stone. (animal-rights activists, please don't write to complain, you know what I mean). On the other hand, I am suspicious of multi-hyphen products. What do you mean, you clean, exfoliate, moisturise and do all my ironing? There's always a niggling feeling that nothing can really be that brilliant, especially when their functions seem unrelated. So what, I hear you ask, is this dual-functioning product doing here? Well, indulge me for a minute. It all began two days into a week-long work trip. I got to my hotel room, had a quick nap and then, on waking, decided that I would wash my hair before going out to dinner that night. At that point, I realised I had left my shampoo at home. This, as any woman of colour knows, is justifiable cause for a major Mariah-level meltdown. It's not like I could just borrow some shampoo from my Caucasian colleagues. I had packed this cleanser at the last minute to use on my body, but as I was desperate, I used it on my hair. And WOW. It was incredible. I had expected to overcompensate for the crunchy hair I'd be left with by overloading it with styling products until I was reunited with my beloved shampoo, but my hair was incredibly soft and pliable post wash. It has coconut and tamanu oils to help restore moisture balance, a cleansing system that removes chlorine, salt and product build-up, and a beautiful tropical scent (neroli and ylang ylang essential oils). It was so good, in fact, that I didn't need to use a conditioner. It hasn't totally restored my faith in the concept of multi-tasking beauty products – they are not all made equal – but this is one I definitely trust.

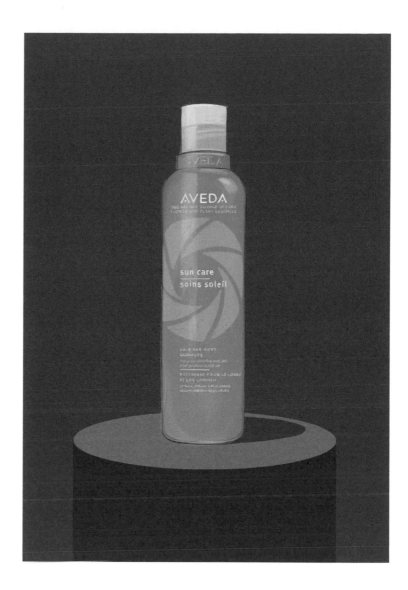

BRIOGEO
Be Gentle, Be Kind™
Avocado + Quinoa Co-Wash

In my experience, most cleanser-conditioners have no slip, do not clean and do not foam. (Yes, I am one of those who, through years of steady indoctrination, loves a sud.) Briogeo's superfood version, however, is easily one of the best I have ever used. This 'clean beauty' brand, founded by Nancy Twine, a brilliant African American who used to work in finance, doesn't target a specific ethnicity. It is all-inclusive and fabulous for natural textured hair. A 4-in-1 marvel, full of oils, vitamins and antioxidants, it cleans, conditions, nourishes and detangles. I expected it to be creamy, nourishing and smell divine. It does smell beautiful (the avocado is not overwhelming), and it is really creamy – however yes, that does mean it doesn't foam (gah). But I needn't have doubted its cleaning abilities. This leaves your hair blissfully clean without stripping it and you don't need to use a conditioner afterwards. The softness and defined curl pattern that follows is so mind blowing, I am rethinking my obsession with foam. Now, this is not a 'one dollop cleans all' situation. You need quite a bit of product so rinse hair vigorously beforehand – particularly if you have a lot of build-up – otherwise you risk using the entire bottle. That is more of a caveat than a gripe, because I have no complaints. Why would I? My hair now moves with the grace of a ballet dancer and shines like a diamond.

CURLSMITH®
Curl Quenching
Conditioning Wash

Coincidence, perhaps, but at the time I discovered this brand – it describes itself as gourmet haircare – I had also been sent, by various brands, products I was assured were 'great for curly or frizzy hair'. While I appreciate people think, somewhat erroneously, this shows they are tailoring their products to my hair texture, I am amazed how many people still think any product that fights the frizz equates to 'perfect for Afro hair'. That can be really frustrating, and there are only so many conversations you can have to try and educate people that the curls on the head of my Irish friend and those sprouting from the scalp of one whose heritage is the deep south of Nigeria, are not quite the same. I was expecting the same level of disappointment and annoyance from this product line, but I was wrong.

I was immediately struck by the nostalgic but modern-looking aesthetic. In a sea of minimalist packaging (which I love but admit can be quite austere at times), it felt novel and interesting. I noticed it was also 'handmade', vegan and 'clean' (paraben-, silicone- and mineral-oil-free). It was developed with a 'community' of trichologists, beauty insiders, bloggers (with varying hair types) and hairstylists, and the wealth of input shows: it is amazing. In fact, I fell so hard for this wash I began gifting it to friends. As a young child, I had found the way Comfort softened clothes fascinating. And so, one day, I unravelled my fresh cornrows and poured half a bottle of fabric softener on my hair, hoping for the same results. My parents went mad. I realised what I expected (from the fabric softener) was the kind of softness this wash delivers. It is so incredibly softening and hydrating; it detangles, adds shine and cleans without killing your hair. This is all down to an impressive array of ingredients that includes andiroba (a hair-nourishing superfood fruit from the Amazon rainforest), shea butter, resurrection flower (known for its remarkable moisture-retention properties), avocado and organic coconut. The shade is silvery white with the texture of a high-quality Greek yogurt (trust me, there's a difference). It is sulphate free, so totally foamless, which would normally gall me, but if you don't have a significant product build-up, it cleans quickly and efficiently. So, there you have it, a curly-girl hair cleanser that actually works on coily girls.

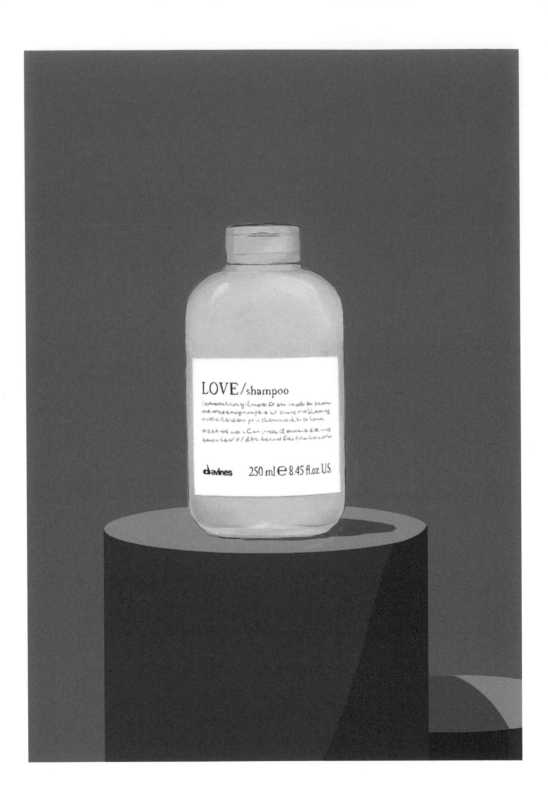

DAVINES
Love Curl Shampoo

Most hair brands tout their curly products as non-discriminatory, that is, they work just as well on a Greek girl's ringlets as they would on 4c girl. Lies, people, lies. The majority of these products fail miserably on Afro hair. This shampoo, however, is EPIC. It works beautifully. The name is pretty apt, and I am totally in love with it, because it really does love curls. It is like washing your hair with an expensive silky perfume – it's a green citrus – that has the texture of a soft, luscious crème. As with all the best shampoos, you don't need very much. It is not suds free, but that is not necessarily an indication of any sinister ingredients; you would be hard-pressed to find a brand so steeped in its conscious ethos I doubt very much that it has compromised on the formulation. The key ingredient in this is a 'Super' Noto almond extract, which is full of healthy fats and proteins to hydrate, moisturise and strengthen the hair. The softening effect is immediate; your hair suddenly melts when it comes into contact with the shampoo – the reaction akin to a teenager suddenly catching sight of her crush and going weak at the knees. You'll find this shampoo doesn't tangle hair (I've used some that have literally given me dreadlocks); instead it loosens curls and separates them. I always like to use a conditioner, but if you find yourself pressed for time, your hair won't be left looking and feeling cornflake-crunchy. It is not high-street prices, but I do think, for such quality, it is great value, leaving you with silky, shiny curls that pop, as opposed to a frizzy mass. I am infatuated. You will be, too.

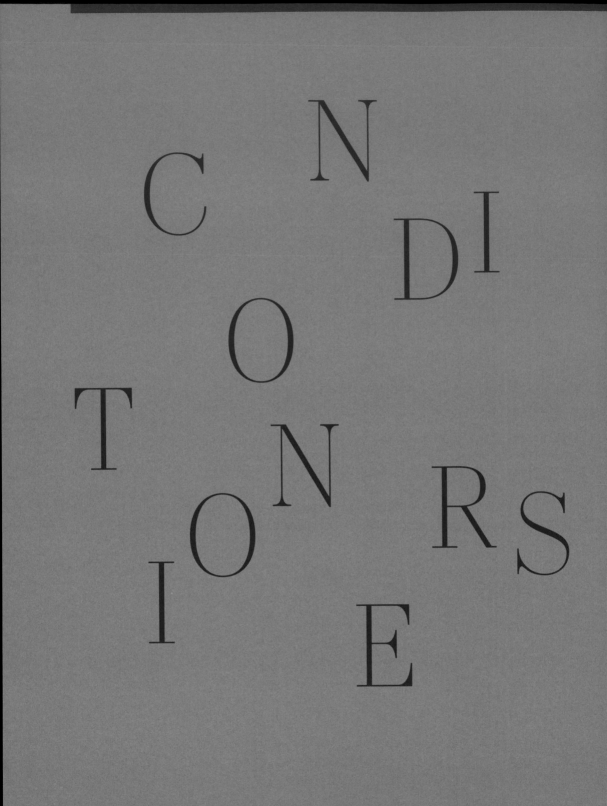

CONDITIONERS

THINGS TO NOTE...

It is worth investing in a home
hair steamer. Your conditioners
and treatments will be much more
efficacious under this. It beats
stuffing your hair into a plastic bag,
wrapping round a hot towel and
feeling the residue dripping down
your back while watching Netflix.

IGK
Hot Girls Hydrating
Conditioner

Sometimes I feel quite conflicted about this brand. On the one hand, I love that cool, Insta-loved rock-and-roll thing it has going on. I love that its marketing is clever, its packaging is standout, and the products have names like Bad & Bougie, Prenup and Rich Kid. But, on the other hand, I look at the narrative of the brand, the Instagram feed, the kind of girls embodied in the campaign, the influencers used to market the products; it is all very, very, how do I say this? ... specific. I mean, I get that the clients are essentially the aforementioned type of woman, and so they developed a brand to meet the needs of this particular type of client. I get that. It kind of makes sense. At the same time, in this age of inclusivity, building a brand around that specific female aesthetic seems somewhat retrograde. And then there's the name Hot Girls – I doubt the founders see this as anything deeper than simple marketing. And yet, beyond all the above, is a boundary-pushing brand with brilliantly formulated products. Of course, not everything in the range is for Afro hair – I mean, dry shampoo? But this conditioner? I'll go as far as to say it is absolutely one of the best I have ever used. I am a sucker for any hair product that pushes the hydration factor, and this definitely does not disappoint. Both the texture (a yellowy-creamy luxe finish), and the scent (guava, coconut water, pink lotus, midnight violet and vanilla) are awesome. The softness and shine this imparts to my hair is insane. It detangles brilliantly, melting away tangles and knots, even without a brush, and curls are deeply moisturised, shiny and defined afterwards. And that's the dilemma: marvellous product; 'You can't sit with us' marketing. Interestingly, the online blurb does say this conditioner is also for 'coily hair'. Which is great. I just wish its inclusiveness was a little more obvious. I guess they could always change the name to Hot Gyals. I joke. But you see my point.

PANTENE
Gold Series Moisture Boost Conditioner

Just like the shampoo in this range, I first encountered this conditioner in a completely blank tester bottle. I tried it out and was immediately addicted. What was this creamy, beautifully but not overbearingly scented thing of wonder? I loved it so much that I found myself looking forward to my hair-washing ritual just so I could use it. It softens – like really, really softens – hydrates and helps repair dry and damaged hair. And you can feel the difference straight away. It has set the bar so high that I had to whittle down the original list of conditioners I had planned to include in this book. Yes, there are many good conditioners out there, but what I have discovered is that the results barely last beyond the bathroom. This, on the other hand, has longevity: your hair still feels soft for days afterwards. It is easily the best affordable conditioner I have used. I often inwardly cringe when I am asked for a specific recommendation, and the product I am recommending is expensive.

Yes, there are some products for which there is no cheaper alternative, but if I have the opportunity to recommend a good value product then I will throw it at as many people as possible. Another thrilling thing is the story behind this, involving ten years of research and more than 3,000 people across continents (from South America to Africa); with the brains behind it (predominantly female) PhD-qualified people of colour. There's something so gratifying about using a product that had you in mind from the start, and not just as an afterthought. Of course, it's not all altruistic – there's money to be made. Still, it makes a change from attending hair-product launches where the texture of my hair is so alien to the brand, I may as well have okra growing out of my scalp.

PHILIP KINGSLEY
Moisture Extreme
Conditioner

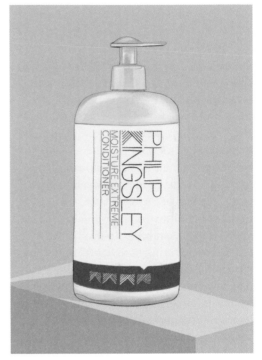

I get that it's not the most exciting-looking product. But this old schooler has been 'doing hair' long before the new kids on the block were a glimmer in their founder's eye. You see Philip Kingsley was the most lauded trichologist in the beauty industry (he has since passed away and the mantle of the brand has been handed down to his daughter, also a trichologist). The beauty of the brand is that it is respected, efficacious, and it's not all about how great it looks on Instagram – the company would rather invest its money and time in making products that don't make your hair fall out. When I first began working in magazines, I ignored the majority, if not all, of the hair products that landed in our office. They were not 'for' me, and they made no bones about it. After a while, of course, I started trying out some of the products, because, you know, that's my job. Which is when I discovered this, a mainstream conditioner that targeted non-Caucasian hair – relaxed and natural. So many people (including hairstylists who break out in a sweat at the thought of handling Afro hair – you know who you are) assume non-Caucasian hair is 'tough', but it is actually fragile and susceptible to breakage. We need a lot of moisture and hydration.

This conditioner does exactly that: it hydrates the hair excellently (particularly when used in a steam treatment), making it noticeably shinier, deeply conditioned and smooth. Now if you are looking for really exacting curl definition, you are probably barking up the wrong tree. However, your hair will have bounce and volume, and the cream formulation – a blend of almond, wheatgerm, avocado and babassu oils – won't weigh down your hair or suffocate your pores. I think that's a pretty fair deal.

DAVINES
Love Conditioner

Despite it being housed in what looks like a takeaway tub (I rather like the simplicity of it), I am smitten with this conditioner. In fact, every time I pick it up I sigh deeply like a delirious, lovesick teenager. The green-citrus smell is addictive – I have to refrain from sniffing it all day. And the effect on my hair, well, it is just awesome. There are so many conditioners on the market that in order to get your hair to a place where it doesn't feel stringy or strawlike, you basically have to engulf it in half the bottle. Not this. And just as well because it is quite a small pot. The impact is pretty immediate. Your hair feels incredibly smooth and soft – the magic ingredient is the olive extract (a hair strengthener

with intense moisturising properties) from Mr Messina's farm, Ficarra, Messina, Italy. No, I have no idea who he is either, but Davines are very transparent about where everything comes from, so this info is written on the packaging. Other ingredients include vitamin E, which also works as an antioxidant to protect hair from the elements, and panthenol, which gives added moisture and shine. Together they provide a certain elasticity – detangling becomes a breeze, you can just use your fingers – and your curls are totally separated. And that is the pièce de résistance: the curl definition. Like an enthusiastic Lycra-clad *Fame* dancer, your curls will be bouncy, stretchy, shiny and happy. Bliss.

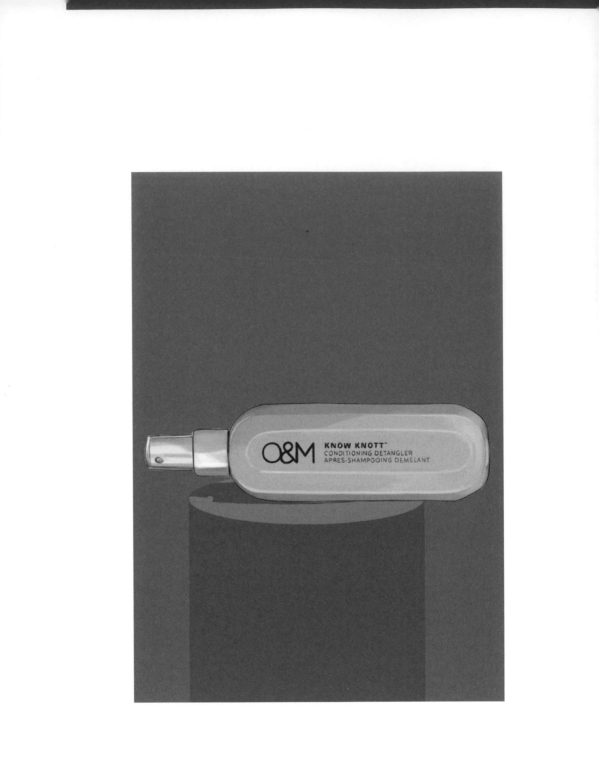

ORIGINAL & MINERAL
Know Knott™ Conditioning Detangler

When I first went natural, it was an utter nightmare. I had a daily tug of war with the idea of going back to chemical relaxers aka the creamy crack. I just didn't understand my hair. I didn't understand this new look, this new feel. I didn't understand why my hair wouldn't react to products the way it normally would. I had spent years becoming an expert at frying my hair – I owned irons and tongs in every barrel size, for every eventuality – and was constantly called on by friends and family members to sort out theirs. I was a regular fixture in the black-hair shops, telling total strangers what weave brand to buy and the best moisturiser to use prior to frying your hair. And now? I had no idea about hair. And it was disconcerting; I even began to dread washing my hair (which now is one of my favourite pastimes – yes, really). So I started to watch a slew of those hair-blogger videos, but I wasn't interested in doing anything fancy with my hair – I didn't have the time, inclination or the upper-arm strength, for that matter,

to spend hours every week doing a twist-out using a million and one products. All I wanted was a product to stop my hair resembling Shredded Wheat, and so far nothing was working. And then this landed at my door, and it changed everything. I'm not quite sure how or why but this peachy-scented spray managed to thoroughly hydrate, soften, detangle and moisturise my hair in one fell swoop. It was phenomenal. Interestingly, it has coconut, argan and macadamia-nut oils in it, all ingredients included in other formulas I had used but had made no difference to my hair – hence I always argue that a good product is not just about ingredients; the efficacy is in the formulation. And what a great formulation this is. I'd go as far as to say it is one of the best detanglers I have used. If not the best. Despite being around for ages, this Australian brand is still under the radar and not as widely available as it deserves. At the time of writing I noticed it had sold out in quite a few places. So, if you do come across it, stock-pile.

DAVINES
Nounou Hair Mask

A few years ago, one of my colleagues on the fashion desk came to me slightly flustered. She was going off on holiday, Nounou hair mask had sold out at her usual outlet, and she needed it TODAY. Help, her eyes pleaded. I managed to get hold of one for her that afternoon. I chuckled to myself as I often do at these ridiculous 'it's the end of the world' champagne problems, but I was also intrigued that a hair mask could do this to a woman. So, of course, I had to use it. And then it made sense. If you are struggling with dry, brittle hair, this is manna from heaven. The foodie theme carries through. Like a lot of Davines products, it comes in a no-frills 'takeaway' tub. The whipped texture – it's got a lot of olive butter and jojoba oil in it to soften and moisturise the hair – looks as if it could have been concocted and dispatched from the kitchen. And the other key ingredient is tomato extract. Now if, like me, you sometimes struggle with gourmand beauty (unless you're a cake, I don't see why you'd want to smell like chocolate or vanilla), this is not one to be concerned about. It won't make you heave; in fact, it smells amazing. The scent is more tomato vine than fruit,

so your hair smells more fresh green scent than pot of stew. The first time I used it, my hair had taken a beating (harsh weather + intense deadlines + minimal upkeep = Miss Havisham's long-lost black sister). Straight away, my hair (aka a big bush of Brillo pads) felt much softer. And that was me simply using it as you would a conditioner, which, in some ways, is cheating because, of course, it is a hair mask. But, let's be honest, who always has time to use a hair mask? The reality is there will be days (many, many days), when you just can't be arsed. Saying that, the best way to use this is as a hair mask – ideally, within a steam treatment. If you have an obliging stylist, take it in and use it in a salon. Otherwise, use it under a home steamer, which you can buy cheaply on Amazon. The results are amazing – intensely moisturising and adds incredible body. Few things to note: be sparing, you don't need much. That said, it's a small tub so don't expect it to last for ever, especially if you have really thick, long hair. And stock up when you can – it's constantly sold out. Once you start using it, you'll understand why my fashion friend behaved like an addict with withdrawal symptoms.

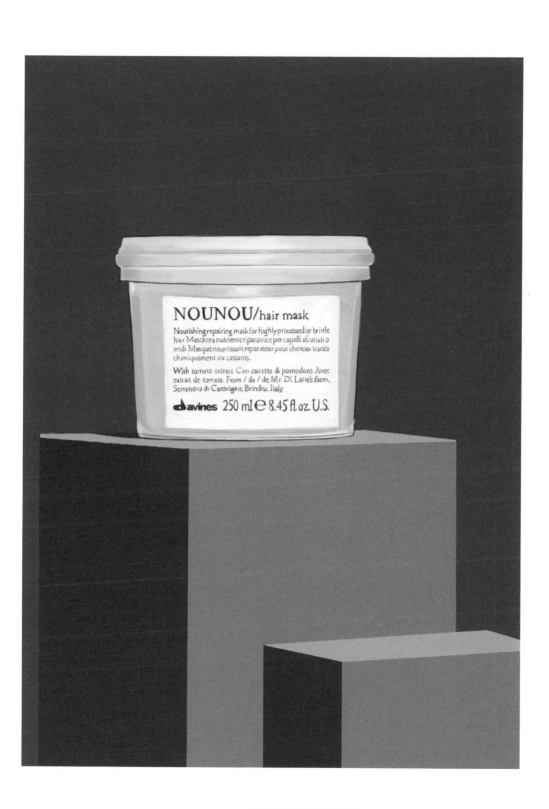

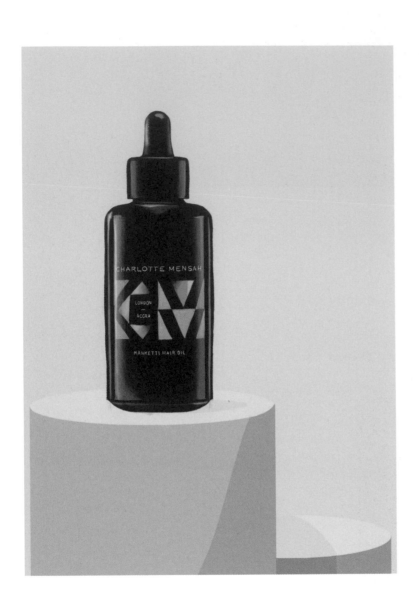

CHARLOTTE MENSAH
Manketti Hair Oil

I had no idea what manketti oil was either until I met Charlotte – the UK's foremost (multi-award-winning) hairstylist for textured hair. Sometimes used interchangeably with mongongo, it's the oil that comes from the nuts of the manketti tree and has incredible emollient and antioxidant properties. This enables hair to survive and remain moisturised and hydrated in extreme temperatures (perfect for British weather). Oils, however, can be tricky. The worst kind can clog the pores on your scalp and around your face (hello, breakouts). And then some simply sit on top of your (now lank) hair strands like a greasy oppressor. The great thing with this is that it does a lot of things you don't expect oils to do. It isn't greasy, it penetrates into the hair as opposed to simply coating it, and I have not experienced any breakouts from using it. That said, when you use it as a hair treatment, the results are far more tangible. The first time I tried it was a number of years ago at Charlotte's Notting Hill salon. When I walked in, my hair needed resurrecting from the dead – the joys of winter – and a decent cut (Charlotte's the one who taught me that if hair has a good shape/cut, everything automatically looks better and she's right). Post wash, Charlotte applied this oil and put me under the steamer, then 20 minutes later, she rinsed it out and blow-dried my hair. When I felt my hair, it was soft, smooth, shiny, hydrated and had incredible movement. Yes, it is quite pricey (you can, however, get the travel size to see if it works for you before committing), but if you use it as part of a monthly treatment as opposed to showering it on daily like a rapper with a bottle of champagne, it should last a while. Also, although it doesn't weigh the hair down, it is definitely heavy for someone with really fine hair, so if that's you, a few drops under a steamer are infinitely better. Then there's the smell – slightly sweet, nutty and clove-like. Tons of people are obsessed with it (so much so that Charlotte has created a candle in the same scent for the cult following). Still, I think it is polarising. Many people find it a little too strong and slightly masculine. Again, it's less potent if not used directly. Whatever the case, it is absolutely worth it. You will have softer, shinier, smoother and less frazzled hair – everything mine wasn't before I walked into Charlotte's salon.

SAHARA SINGLE BIBLE
Soft Oil Organic
Hair Softener

The brilliant Museum of Brands in London explores how consumerism has shaped the world since Victorian times. So, for anyone who grew up in the UK, it is a real nostalgia hit – expect to see throwbacks to your childhood: Game Boys, Candy cigarettes, *Just Seventeen* magazine (yes, I know, for some people this is going completely over your head – just go with it). If the museum were also to reflect the evolving haircare arsenal of the black community, this oil (along with Blue Magic – yes, it's blue – and Luster's Pink Oil Moisturizer – yes, it's pink) would have pride of place. It is not extinct by any means (you won't find it in many modern bathroom cabinets, but you can still find it in black-hair shops), but it is quite vintage. It's like an old friend you see every few years: you've long fled the confines of a small town you both grew up in. You, now a city girl with a fancy, frenetic lifestyle. She, on the other hand, never left her parochial environs and doesn't quite fit in with your new friends. But you catch up from time to time, and it's lovely. Which sums up my relationship with this dense, syrupy, gooey oil. It is not the most fashionable oil. It does not have the weightlessness of its modern counterparts. Its scent – a combination of aloe vera (single bible is the Jamaican term for this plant), rosemary and tea tree – smells more like something you would use to treat insect bites. Polarising? Absolutely. But surely I can't be the only one who loves that medicated scent. Also the key purpose of this oil is to deal with hair and scalp problems – you know, all the really unsexy aspects of haircare (like dandruff, itchiness and flakiness) that everyone pretends never happen. And the bottle: it looks like something time forgot. So why am I recommending it? Well, I have found that when I dealt with post-baby hair loss this was the brilliant stimulant – you need just a teeny bit – that coaxed my hair back to life. When my scalp is feeling out of sorts, this oil is the tranquillity it needs. And when used in a steam treatment, the softness you get afterwards is unbeatable. But, yes, there is the texture to contend with: it is as thick as honey; so fine-haired girls should go easy. And if you hate the smell of antiseptic, you may struggle. But ask yourself this: would I really struggle with a product that promotes hair growth and makes my hair softer than the fluffy insides of a fresh doughnut? I know the answer to that.

SUNNY ISLE
Rosemary Jamaican Black Castor Oil

Take one look at the 'oil' aisle in any black-hair shop, and unless you know exactly what you are looking for, it's enough to make you want to lie down in a dark room. Lime oil, wonder oil, olive oil, mustard oil, custard oil. OK, no, I haven't seen custard oil, but I put that in to see if you are still paying attention. Out of the oils, the two I have found to work well on hair are rosemary and castor. However, what I have also learnt is that the quality of the oils can be the difference between a cubic zirconia and a rare diamond. So many of the oils on sale have either been blended with other cheaper oils or the key ingredient just isn't high enough in strength or quality. Sunny Isle, for me, is the most authentic. Its castor oil is a really thick, unctuous dark oil. While you might be tempted to run a mile, please don't. Castor oil is an incredible humectant, so it is great for locking in moisture. It also reduces inflammation, which helps with any scalp issues. Rosemary is equally brilliant, known for stimulating hair growth. So you take the best quality of these ingredients, combine them, and what you are left with is a powerhouse. Like most of these thick oils, applying directly to equally thick, dense hair is fine. Fine hair, not so much. Either way, it's worth going easy on it, otherwise you end up with dust-attracting hair that you'll need to wash ridiculously regularly – and with half a bottle of shampoo each time. I prefer to use it within a fortnightly deep-steam treatment. Massage it into your scalp and hair post wash, and you will revolutionise the condition of your hair and notice that it's much more hydrated, supple, shiny and full. Do bear in mind that the dark castor oil does stain, so save your 400-thread-count, off-white linen for another time in your life. Please note, you won't see the results straight away, so it might feel like you're watching your phone for a text response from your most recent date. Your date might never come back to you, but I bet your hairline will.

STYLING

THINGS TO NOTE...

Any naturalista should always have
a great detangler to hand – it will
change your hair and your life. All
heavy styling products are also hair
changing, although not in a good way;
so choose wisely. Milky textures are
a brilliant non-greasy halfway house
between lotions and butters. Not all
gels are terrible.

TEXTURE MY WAY®
Easy Comb Leave-In Detangling & Softening Crème Therapy

First things first, it would be nice if this brand could make its products look a little bit different from each other. They look so similar I have on countless occasions almost moisturised my hair with shampoo. I am always on the lookout for great detanglers and have sometimes taken to making my own. This means adding whatever product is within arm's reach (oils, sprays, leave-in conditioners and so on) and mixing them together in a spray bottle with some water – ideally, using bottled water, especially if you live in a hard-water area. The problem with this haphazard product selection, of course, is that I can never remember my 'recipe', so sometimes it's great and other times it's a disaster.

I love this Texture My Way product because it is a moisturiser and a detangler, and it manages to excel at both. A good proportion of the moisturisers for Afro hair usually have some or all of the following issues: they linger on the hair (as opposed to penetrating it), leave a white film, are thick, heavy and greasy or so 'light' they barely touches the sides, even on fine hair. Surprisingly, this product has the right balance. It literally drenches the hair in moisture (shea butter and olive oil) but doesn't leave a sticky residue; it also works across a spectrum of hair types. It says easy comb, and I can testify that it is exactly that: hair is immediately softer and easier to get a comb through knots. It also ticks the clean beauty boxes: no sulphate, no parabens, no petroleum or mineral oils. Yes it's not fragrance-free, but I don't think the floral-meets-citrus scent is such a terrible price to pay for knot-free hair.

AVEDA™ Brilliant™ Emollient Finishing Gloss

This is one of my favourite Aveda hair products. The Brilliant range is the one that is particularly suited to Afro hair. Aveda began championing holistic beauty, diversity and environmental responsibility long before it became fashionable. And, unlike a lot of brands that started in the area of eco-beauty, it actually makes products that are efficacious and not just full of guff. This gloss being one of them. The key ingredient here is rice bran oil, a vitamin- and antioxidant-rich oil that contains omega-3 and omega-6 fatty acids and a high concentration of vitamin E. It is great for softening hair without weighing it down. This divinely scented gel-like oil comes in a small bottle with a pump, so it is dispensed in equally small, controlled measurements. If you like to slather products on to your heart's content, you might find this infuriating, but, to be honest, you don't actually need very much. Consider this the finishing touch for your hair, like the oil sheens of old, except this doesn't punch a hole in the ozone layer every time you use it. And it doesn't drip down your forehead and your neck and your collar and give you acne. And this imparts goodness, too (even protecting hair from UV rays). So there's no need to get carried away with it: the operative word here is 'finishing', so don't use it like you would a moisturiser; think of it as 'decorative', as in a garnish, not the useless figurines our grandmothers used to display on the mantelpiece. I like that you can use this across various hair types and styles – locs, braids, relaxed hair, natural hair – but, of course, you can't please everyone. One criticism I hear is that it is a little pricey for the size, which is fair enough. But before you think you can simply rush out to Brixton market to buy rice bran oil by the gallon, do remember that is only one of the ingredients in this. Some people have also said that it doesn't smooth down hair for long. Well, I'll add this: it is not a gel. The priority here is shine and softness, and on that it delivers. And then, of course, as with anything remotely oily, someone always finds it too greasy. Just apply the 'less is more' school of thought, and you'll be fine. And if you are tempted otherwise, hold the gloss in your hand and repeat this line: 'I don't need to asphyxiate my hair to get the shine factor.' There you go. Thought for the Day.

AUNT JACKIE'S™
Tame My Edges
Smoothing Gel

I wear my hair in a super low-maintenance 'dancer's bun', and this is the product I use around my edges. After years of hiding half my face under faux fringes, weaves, pick-and-drop braids, wigs, you name it, I am now obsessed with keeping my hair completely off my face. I wanted to come to terms with my face and no longer use hair as a crutch: I Am Not My Hair, and all that. It is an obsession that has had me contemplating shaving my head on more occasions than I care to remember. But that's another story. So, yes, I love this product because it does a great job – I don't need to pull my hair super tight to slick my hairline back, as this does it all for me. It is a soft, see-through orange gel, that, yes, does feel quite thick and a bit sticky, and not particularly pliable, but the trick is to be really measured. It's almost like good-quality Botox (for the record, I haven't had that myself) for the edges of your hair. It keeps them in place all day, it doesn't harden (that's a no-no for me), doesn't flake (another deal-breaker), and then it wears off but with no side effects. Unlike the gels of old, there is no build-up; my hair feels soft and moisturised, and the recipe – a flaxseed,

argan and grapeseed-oil concoction – strengthens hair while combating thinning, shedding and breakage. Plus I can take it in my handbag. So it's perfect really. And yet I have a bugbear. I am bristled by the word 'tame' in the context of our Afro hair. The words 'combative', 'wiry' and 'unruly' are used to describe our hair type, and it riles me. We have been told for so long that our hair is somehow less than, that it is 'difficult', that it is not good enough, that it is unacceptable in its authentic form, and it must always be wrestled down and 'disciplined' to behave in a way that goes against its natural self. I honestly don't think the brand (or, indeed, other brands) has thought too deeply about this. Not because it is insensitive or ignorant, but because we have all been so conditioned to the normality of these terms that most of the time we don't bat an eyelid. I don't know about you, but I find it jarring to hear brands talking about the 'coarse', 'undisciplined' stuff that grows out of our scalp, like it's something of an aberration. I genuinely do love this brand, but it needs to change its language around our hair. And, if we are being honest, it is probably something we all need to do too.

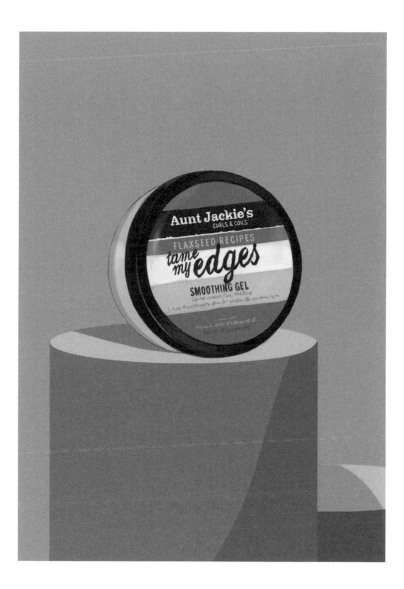

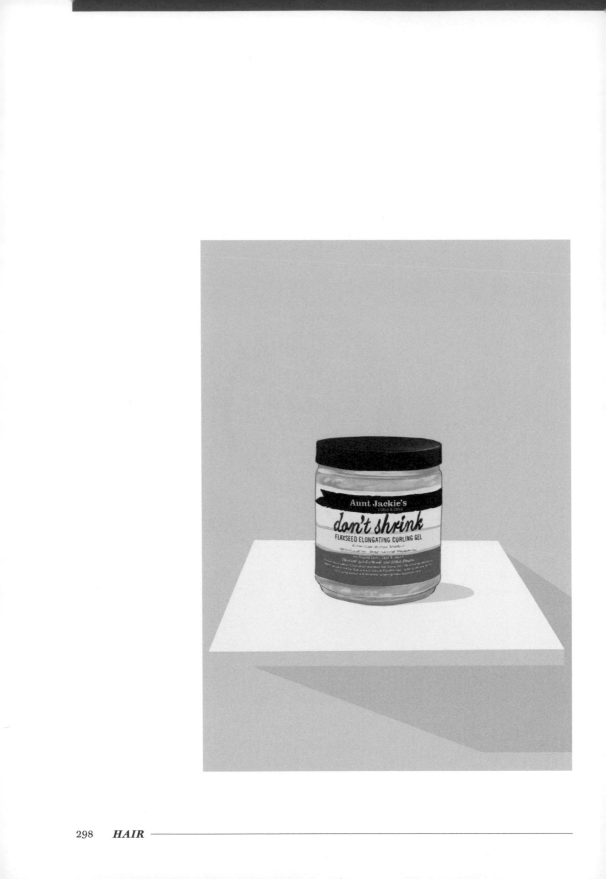

AUNT JACKIE'S™
Don't Shrink Flaxseed
Elongating Curling Gel

Oh, my goodness, shrinkage. It really is a thing, isn't it? During the time I was learning about my new natural hair (mostly spent looking in the mirror, shrieking, 'WHO ARE YOU?!'), I learnt about this thing called 'shrinkage'. For those who don't know, it's when your hair looks much shorter than it actually is – the tighter your curl pattern, the more it absorbs moisture, the more it shrinks. Google 'shrinkage Afro hair', and you will get the gist. Be warned: looking at pictures of women demonstrating how their hair has shrunk up to 80 per cent of its actual length – and what it looks like when stretched – is addictive viewing. So, of course, short of (no pun intended) straightening your hair, women are always on the lookout for products that cause minimal shrinkage. I personally found 'shrinkage' meant I couldn't pull my hair back in a bun with ease, and this is where this gel comes in. I did baulk at the idea of using a gel in my hair. I had terrifying visions of hair that would harden like a helmet, with the residue shedding all over my clothes like a

snake with leprosy. But this is a different kind of gel. It doesn't have that harsh injection of sinus-irritating alcohol (this is the key culprit for causing hair to dry out and flake); rather it smells like the inside of a sweetie jar. It is full of moisturising conditioners – flaxseed, olive oil, shea butter and other fatty acids – so it actually has hair-health properties. The texture is watery light and doesn't sit stiffly on your hair like those 1990s rubbery gels. Instead it eases in like a moisturiser, and your hair doesn't harden. You can use it for twists, braid-outs, Bantu knots and curls. I tend to use it post wash; I simply run it through my hair – it gives amazing stretch and shine – then put my hair in a bun. It is my fail-safe, one-stop shop to a Happy Hair day (considering I used to spend my lecture time and student loan at my hair salon, even I'm amazed at how low maintenance I've become). I bulk buy this and share the love; it is, easily, the hair product I recommend the most to women of colour. I can't promise it will change your life, but I can guarantee it will change your hair.

DAVINES
Oi All In One Milk

It was probably around five years ago when a hair perfume first landed on my desk. I recall looking at it, bemused. 'No one's going to buy this,' I scoffed presumptuously. I was wrong. While I wouldn't go as far as to say it has gained mammoth traction, there must be some demand (from people who love buying ridiculous things maybe), because many more brands have launched into this category since. I get that sometimes you just want your hair to smell a little more elevated than a basic shampoo; I get it, but is it worth it? Not when you have something like this hair milk. The smell is utterly marvellous – so much so that many fans use the oil as a scent. Beyond that it offers up some great hair benefits. The key ingredient here is roucou oil, which is found in the rainforest and protects hair from environmental stresses and UV damage. It works as a leave-in conditioner that intensely nourishes hair without weighing it down, which is key for anyone with fine hair. It also works well on thick hair. There is a tendency to assume that because you have thick hair you need more product. Not necessarily. While this is a light conditioner-like formula, don't be overzealous in your application – you don't need half as much as you might think you do. I like to use it post washing, when my hair is still really damp, and then I brush through – it isn't a curl definer, mind you. If I'm feeling indulgent, I'll add some of the oil version of this (it's more expensive, though), and then I'm done. You can use this on dry hair, but I find it much more effective on wet hair – and I am less inclined to use the entire bottle. Either way, it makes your hair smell exquisite, all day long, while also softening, detangling, hydrating and minimising frizz. That's a darn sight more than a hair perfume could hope to achieve.

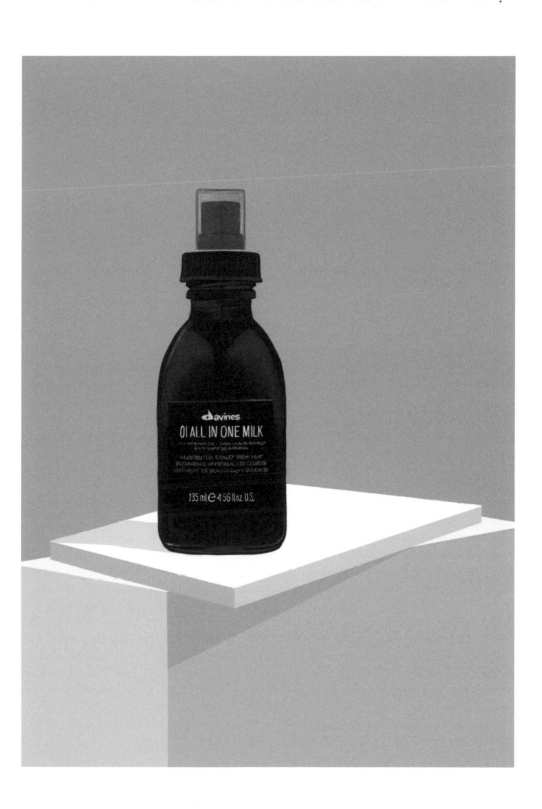

ECO STYLER®
Professional Styling
Gel Krystal

Sometimes, in the rare moments when I have nothing better to do with my time, I find myself wondering whether gels even have a place in modern society. That sounds like such an odd thing to say, but they are so old school, don't you think? I have flashbacks to the years when running out of gel, for me, was a full-blown national crisis. Gels took me through my finger-wave (pasted on my forehead) years. They also aggravated my acne and made my hair hard, crunchy and broken. And, so, I have a weird thing with gels. Which is why it's odd for me that this product is here. But this is a different type of gel. My hair is completely natural but, as I've said before, I don't have the time or even the inclination to experiment with tons of different styles. I feel I have channelled so much energy into experimental hairstyles for so many years (I once admitted that the time I spent on my hair could easily amount to a teenage life) that the desire is now totally spent. And so I've gone to the other extreme. My signature hairstyle, if you will, is a bun with a middle parting. But in order to get my hair into a bun, it needs gel. I knew I didn't want a gel that was a throwback to the crunchy days, I didn't want something that flaked, and I certainly didn't want

something that destroyed my hair health. And here was my answer. This is essentially a water-based, no-alcohol gel that gives my hair stretch and enables me to pull it back in a bun without any tension. I use it as a last step in my hair regime – that is, post wash, detangling, moisturising and so on, and what I'm left with is a high-shine slick bun that stays pretty much perfect for at least a week, after which I wash my hair and start the process over. I don't suggest combing it through the hair. Yes, it is hydrating; no, it is not drying, but, bottom line, it is not a moisturiser, so I would advise you use it in conjunction with a product that deeply conditions. If you look at the side of the tub, you will notice a '10'. There are many variants of this gel in the range. There's one with coconut oil, another with olive oil, another with argan oil and so forth. The scores on the tub indicate their level of hold, '10' being the highest. Your choice of hold depends on your hair type and needs. I have pretty much tried them all; Krystal (10) is the best for slicking back 4c hair. It holds like a superpower but, unlike its contemporaries of old, won't destroy your hair and give you spots. Here you go.

SHEAMOISTURE
Coconut Hibiscus Curl Style Milk

Are you sitting down? OK, because I am going to say something that is quite possibly irreligious in haircare circles. Everyone raves about everything SheaMoisture, but I've yet to find a handful of products from the brand that I really love. There. I've said it. And I can hear the intake of breath. To be fair, my criterion for great haircare products have become harder to fulfil ever since I went natural, so I will admit I am a bit of a tricky customer. I should also mention that SheaMoisture has extensive ranges of products, and I cannot profess to have used every single one of them; so it may well be that I have simply yet to unearth tons of truly game-changing products. Right now I feel I'm in the midst of 'The Emperor's New Clothes'. That said, this hair milk is SUPERB. If your hair is thick and curly and gets really parched, this silky opaque milk is a requisite. There are so many plusses. There's the luscious creamy texture that penetrates deeply into the hair, which is also a softening moisturiser that aids detangling; aids being the operative word here. I wouldn't use it solely as a detangler – it is too thick for that – but it is effective on post-wash damp hair and works considerably well on dry (as in non-wet) hair also. Most moisturisers struggle to do both efficiently. If you choose to use this daily, be sparing – the build-up will dull your hair and make your curls lank. The addition of hibiscus makes the scent less coconutty and more ... floral coconut. Yes, I know there's no such thing as a floral coconut but just go with me on this one.

CURLSMITH®
Moisture Memory Reactivator

There are not many traditional hair moisturisers in here. Fundamentally, the reason for this is that despite the deluge of products you are faced with when you visit a beauty-supply store, the quality and the efficacy of many are questionable. They are either heavy oils, which attract dirt and make you look as if you haven't washed your hair in a decade. Or they are so light they do nothing; so you touch your hair, and it still makes the noise of a crushed-up crisp packet. The brands that think about moisturising in terms of hydration and quenching a thirst are coming up with products that work. Like this one. The name is a bit confusing; not because it doesn't make sense, but because we are so used to putting things into traditional categories that when something doesn't say 'moisturiser', 'conditioner' or 'shampoo', we are like, What the hell are you? So just view this as one of the new genre of category-fluid products. The point of it is to extend the life of your hair between washes – like our Caucasian counterparts do with dry shampoo.

Except there is nothing drying about this. Ingredients include avocado, andiroba, aloe vera, apricot, resurrection flower and rosemary, which all help to soften, lock in moisture and promote hair growth. You can use this as a leave-in conditioner, post-wash, as a moisturiser between washes, as a refresher boost twist-outs or a thirst-quencher for days when your hair has spent too much time in the sun. The texture, a water-light serum in spray form, means your hair never feels overwhelmed. I would recommend it to all natural-hair women, it's fabulous.

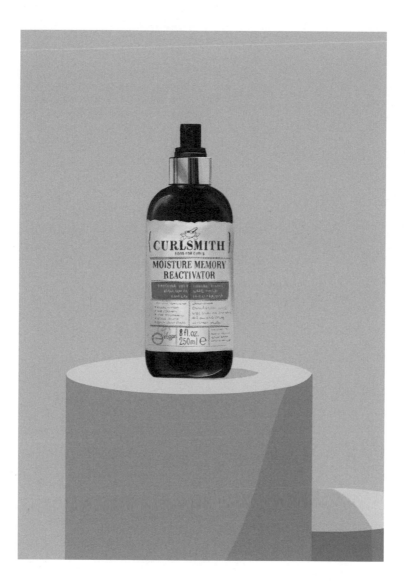

When I mentioned to a few people that I was writing a book on products suitable for women of colour, they were doubtful that I would find enough to fill even a quarter of this book.

As I come to the end of *Palette*, I am rather smug that I have proved them wrong. There are close to 200 products in here, all of which I have personally tried and loved and included in my edit. Of course this is not an exhaustive compilation. There are new brands, products and new discoveries (for me at least) every day. It was, and is, impossible to include them all. There are many that did not make the cut because I felt there was a superior alternative. Then there were some that didn't make it in due to logistical factors I won't bore you with. A few standouts include **Antidote Street**, a brilliant site catering to Afro and textured hair. It sells some really cool, independent (and many black-owned) brands such as **Dizziak**, **Jim + Henry** and **Anita Grant**. **MDM Flow** by Florence Adepoju creates hip-hop inspired lipsticks with incredible pigments and Sherrille Riley of **Beauty Edit Mayfair** is developing great 'all-inclusive' brow products that push the boundaries of technology.

The number of beauty products available to women of colour is growing and it is heartening to be able to celebrate them in *Palette*. That said, if I'm being honest, this book isn't really about beauty. It is about representation and being treated equally. While there have been positive movements in the industry, I still come across brands that purposely will not extend their shade range past the pale because they don't believe we are a relevant part of their customer base. What makes this even more problematic is that a global, highly influential retailer sees no issue with actively seeking out and stocking brands that, through their actions, have completely disregarded an entire demographic. There are huge retailers that take on black-owned brands (with a product line that caters to all nationalities) and yet, like the ultimate backhanded compliment, decide to only stock them in 'ethnic areas' because they don't believe it will sell in their more centrally-located stores. The ridiculous insinuation being that people of colour only live and shop in certain areas. I know of retailers who have round-the-houses conversations – I'm talking years – about stocking what they deem as 'black brands' and yet never put their money where their mouth is because they are, ultimately, not willing to take a chance on a brand that speaks to anything other than what they consider to be the mainstream. There are so many more stories that serve as proof that, although we have made some gloriously exciting strides, there is further ground to break, there are minds that still need to be broadened and there are bigger, deeper and more uncomfortable conversations to be had. For real change to take place, many of these will have to go deeper than extending shades of foundations beyond 'Biscuit'.

THANKS

Writing a book is like giving birth. The process can be lengthy and painful and there are (many) moments you rue the day you believed it was a good idea. In times like this, you need human epidurals. I had a few. Emma Paterson, thank you for being a kind, encouraging and all-round utterly brilliant agent. The Hodder team: Melissa Cox, your relentless enthusiasm, belief in this book and endless patience with me (!) has kept my head above water. I once read somewhere that 'Perseverance is the hard work you do after you get tired of doing the hard work you already did'. Thank you, Melissa, for helping me to persevere. Lily, I am so grateful for your tireless work and for cracking the whip in the most gracious way. Alice, you know I wouldn't have a clue what to do with InDesign and yet you indulge my very vocal thoughts and ideas on layouts, design and fonts. Thank you. Jasmine, your excitement for this book is wonderfully contagious – thank you for your 'let's reach for the skies' ethos. Spiros, thank you for your beautiful illustrations.

To Michelle Obama's *Becoming*, David Sedaris' *Calypso* and Sally Rooney's *Normal People*. You all provided my breath of fresh prose when I needed a break from talking about exfoliating dead skin and matte lipsticks that won't turn your lips into prunes.

To Edward Enninful, thank you for being an inspiration and championing this book, and Lisa Eldridge for being so supportive.

To all the women, on social media and IRL, who approach me for beauty recommendations. You are a constant reminder that this book needed to be written.

To my sisters, daughter and mum (aka HRH) thank you for rolling up your sleeves to organise my 'research' (i.e. millions of beauty products) just so I wouldn't drown in them. To my amazing father for teaching me to believe for more.

Thank you Emma North for being such a brilliant assistant.

To YR and the boys, I know that me being MIA while trying to hit deadline was not always convenient. Thank you; words could never be enough.

To God. Thank you for showing me 'All things are possible to those who believe'. (Mark 9:23)

INDEX